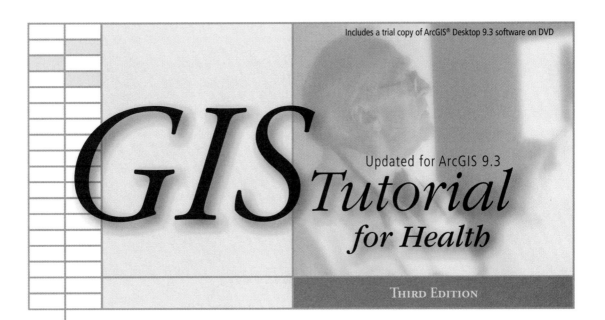

Includes a trial copy of ArcGIS® Desktop 9.3 software on DVD

GIS Tutorial

Updated for ArcGIS 9.3

for Health

THIRD EDITION

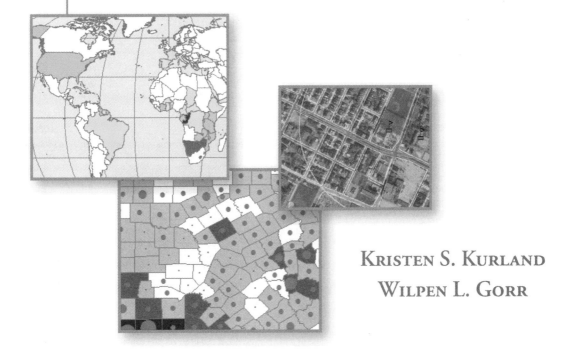

KRISTEN S. KURLAND

WILPEN L. GORR

ESRI PRESS
REDLANDS, CALIFORNIA

Esri Press, 380 New York Street, Redlands, California 92373-8100

Copyright © 2006–2007, 2009 Esri
All rights reserved. First edition 2006. Second edition 2007. Third edition 2009

14 13 12 11 10   2 3 4 5 6 7 8 9 10

Printed in the United States of America

Library of Congress Cataloging-in-Publication Data
Kurland, Kristen Seamens, 1966–
       GIS tutorial for health / Kristen S. Kurland, Wilpen L. Gorr.—3rd ed., updated for ArcGIS 9.3
          p.   cm.
Includes bibliographical references.
       ISBN 978-1-58948-224-1 (pbk. : alk. paper)
       1. Medical geography—Data processing. 2. Geographic information systems. 3. ArcGIS. I. Gorr, Wilpen L. II. Title.
       [DNLM: 1. ArcGIS. 2. Geographic Information Systems—Programmed Instruction. 3. Topography, Medical—Programmed Instruction.
       W 18.2 K96g 2009]
       RA792.G67   2009
       614.4'20285—dc22   2008051417

Ask for Esri Press titles at your local bookstore or order by calling 1-800-447-9778. You can also shop online at www.esri.com/esripress. Outside the United States, contact your local Esri distributor.

Esri Press titles are distributed to the trade by the following:

In North America:
Ingram Publisher Services
Toll-free telephone: (800) 648-3104
Toll-free fax: (800) 838-1149
E-mail: customerservice@ingrampublisherservices.com

In the United Kingdom, Europe, Middle East and Africa, Asia, and Australia:
Eurospan Group
3 Henrietta Street
London WC2E 8LU
United Kingdom
Telephone: 44(0) 1767 604972
Fax: 44(0) 1767 601640
E-mail: eurospan@turpin-distribution.com

Contents

Acknowledgments

We would like to thank all who made this book possible.

GIS Tutorial for Health was used by students at Carnegie Mellon University before it went to ESRI Press for publication. During this time, the students and teaching assistants who used the book provided us with significant feedback. Their thoughtful comments guided our revisions and helped improve the content and overall quality of this book.

We are very grateful to the many individuals, organizations, and vendors who have generously supplied us with interesting GIS cases and data, including Dr. Bruce Dixon, Gerald Barron, Jo Ann Glad, Dr. LuAnn Brink, Glenda Christy, Dan Cinpinski, Mike Diskin, Bruce Good, Dave Namey, and Thom Stulginski of the Allegheny County Health Department; Ross Capaccio of röös design + consulting, and Thom D. Freyer, CAE of the American College of Healthcare Executives, for the datasets used in the "Partners for Success" chapter deployment project; Carl Kinkade of the Centers for Disease Control and Prevention (CDC); Noel S. Zuckerbraun, MD, MPH, assistant professor of pediatrics, Department of Pediatrics, Division of Pediatric Emergency Medicine, Children's Hospital of Pittsburgh, University of Pittsburgh School of Medicine; Barbara A. Gaines, MD, director, Benedum Trauma Program, assistant professor of surgery, Children's Hospital of Pittsburgh, University of Pittsburgh School of Medicine; Noor Ismail, Mike Homa, and Lena Andrews of the City of Pittsburgh, Department of City Planning; The Trustees of Dartmouth College, The Dartmouth Atlas of Health Care (*www.dartmouthatlas.org*); Linda Williams Pickle, PhD, and David Stinchcomb of the National Cancer Institute, The Cancer Mortality Maps & Graph Web site (*http://www3.cancer.gov/atlasplus/index.html*); Chris Chalmers, GIS coordinator, Nebraska Health and Human Services, Bioterrorism Response Section director for GIS Public Health Research, University of Nebraska-Lincoln, CALMIT; Maurie Kelly of Pennsylvania Spatial Data Access (PASDA); U.S. Geological Survey and U.S. Census Bureau; Tele Atlas for use of their USA datasets contained within the ESRI Data & Maps 2004 Media Kit.

Finally, thanks to the entire team at ESRI, especially Bill Davenhall, Ann Bossard, Seth Waife, Peggy Harper, Laura Bowden, Kerri Manorek, and the production and editing staff at ESRI Press, including Claudia Naber, Michael Law, Tiffany Wilkerson, Donna Celso, and Jay Loteria.

Preface

GIS Tutorial for Health is a unique textbook for teaching GIS to health professionals. It embeds learning GIS software in the context of health-care scenarios. While solving real problems, students get many opportunities to visualize and analyze health-related data. Key to this book are its health-care scenarios: they address substantive issues of health care, decision support requirements for policy and planning, and technical requirements of spatial data sources and processing.

Each chapter:

+ *Begins with a health issue or problem that has a spatial component.* Learning a new tool or software package works best in the context of work that is interesting to you. So, we begin by stating a health issue or problem that can be better understood or solved using GIS.

+ *Follows with a conceptual section on the solution approach.* This section provides knowledge and principles on underlying GIS methods. When learning and applying GIS, you often need general knowledge to understand specific steps and workflows. Whenever possible, we have separated such material into brief descriptions preceding the tutorial of a chapter. As a result, you can read this material before sitting down at a computer.

+ *Has a step-by-step tutorial to carry out the solution using ArcGIS.* Each section of the tutorial has numbered steps and corresponding screen captures along with user dialogs and resulting outputs. The steps follow workflows that you can use on other projects. Interspersed throughout the tutorial are "Your Turn" exercises that have you repeat lessons just learned. These exercises help you to start internalizing the ArcGIS steps and workflows.

+ *Ends with hands-on exercises that require independent thinking in applying the knowledge and skills gained in the chapter.* By working through these exercises, you will make ArcGIS a reliable and routine tool for your analyses.

Furthermore, the final two chapters of the book each present a relevant case study for you to work through on your own. Each case has a series of requirements, input datasets, structure required for GIS analysis, and maps and reports for you to produce.

The target audience for the book includes health management students and practitioners, computer specialists who want to work in the health field, as well as health-care managers and researchers who want to gain proficiency in GIS. This book serves primarily as a computer lab textbook, but it can also be used for self-study. The beginning chapters of *GIS Tutorial for Health* can be used for short two- to three-day courses.

If you are new to ArcGIS Desktop and are using this book as a self-study guide, we recommend you work through the chapters in order. However, the chapters are largely independent of each other, so you can use them in the order that best fits you or your class's needs.

This book comes with one CD and one DVD. The CD contains data needed to carry out the tutorials, exercises, and case studies. The DVD contains a 180-day trial of ArcGIS 9.3. You will need to install the data and the software to perform the exercises in this book. (If you already have ArcView 9.3, ArcEditor 9.3, or ArcInfo 9.3 installed, you only need to install the data.) Instructions for installing the CD and DVD that come with this book are included in appendix C.

For teacher resources and updates related to this book, go to *www.esri.com/esripress /gistutorialhealth3*.

After teaching GIS for over 15 years, we know that you—like our own students—will enjoy this subject and software. Go to it!

OBJECTIVES

Define GIS
Define spatial data for graphic and image map layers
Review the national infrastructure for spatial data
Review the unique capabilities of GIS
Demonstrate how GIS can be used for health applications
Introduce ArcGIS and its user interface

GIS Tutorial 1

Introducing GIS and health applications

Geographic information systems (GIS) is a technology with unique and valuable applications for policy makers, planners, and managers in many fields, including public health and health care. GIS software and applications enable you to visualize and process data in ways never before possible. The purpose of this book is to provide you with hands-on experience using the premier GIS software package ArcGIS Desktop in the context of health applications. You need not have any previous experience using GIS.

The next section describes GIS, its inputs, and special capabilities, followed by a discussion of health issues and GIS applications. We also preview the upcoming tutorials in this book, then introduce you to ArcGIS software in a short tutorial.

What is GIS?

GIS is a multidisciplinary software system that engages geographers, computer scientists, social scientists, planners, engineers, and others. Consequently, it has been defined from several different perspectives (e.g., see Clarke 2003). We prefer a definition that emphasizes GIS as an information system: *GIS is a system for input, storage, processing, and retrieval of spatial data.* Except for the additional word "spatial," this is a standard definition for an information system. Spatial components include a digital map infrastructure, GIS software with unique functionality based on location, and new mapping applications for organizations of all kinds. Next, we define and discuss these distinctive aspects of GIS.

Spatial data

Spatial data is information about the locations and shapes of geographic features, in the form of either vector or raster data. Graphic maps, also known as vector maps, are created with layers that have features drawn using points, lines, and polygons. Geographic objects have a variety of shapes, but all of them can be represented as one of three geometric forms—a polygon, a line, or a point. A polygon is a closed area with a boundary consisting of connected straight lines. For example, figure 1.1 is a map with two polygon map layers (state and county boundaries), a line layer of rivers, and a point layer of cities with populations of 250,000 or more. The state and county boundaries are coterminous, that is, they share boundaries and do not overlap each other. We used fill color within the county polygons to show the mortality of lung cancer for white males, which has some striking geographic patterns to be discussed later in this tutorial.

Associated with individual point, line, or polygon features are data records that provide identifying and descriptive data attributes. For example, in figure 1.1 the labels for the names of states and cities come from tables of attribute records associated with each map layer. You will revisit this map in the tutorial where you will use ArcGIS to explore map layers and spatial patterns of cancer mortality.

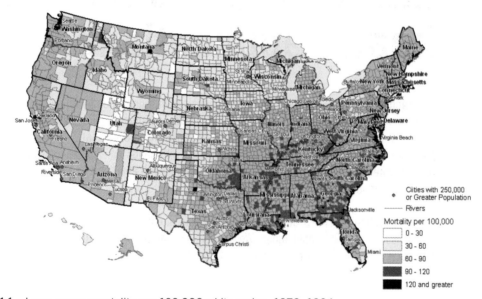

Figure 1.1 Lung cancer mortality per 100,000 white males, 1970–1994.

Sources: (a) ESRI Data & Maps 2005 and (b) The Cancer Mortality Maps and Graph Web site: The National Cancer Institute

Raster maps are aerial photographs, satellite images, or images created with software that are stored in standard digital image formats, such as tagged image file format (TIFF) or Joint Photographic Experts Group (JPEG). An image file is a rectangular array, or raster, of tiny square pixels. Each pixel has a single value and solid color, and corresponds to a small, square area on the ground, from 6 inches to 3 feet on a side for high-resolution images. (Pixels are also often referred to as cells.) Accompanying the image files are world files that provide georeferencing data, including the upper left pixel's location coordinates and the width of each pixel in ground units. The world file provides the data needed, so the GIS software needs to assemble individual raster datasets into larger areas and overlay them with aligned vector datasets.

Viewed on a computer screen or on a paper map, a raster map can provide a detailed backdrop of physical features. In figure 1.2, an aerial photograph overlaid with vector map layers, shows locations where serious injuries of child pedestrians occurred in relation to public playgrounds. The two boundaries surrounding the parks are 1,250- and 2,500-foot buffers used to study injury rates near parks. You will explore the GIS data behind this map in the exercises in this tutorial and then in depth in tutorial 7, where you will create and use buffers similar to those in figure 1.2.

Map layers have geographic coordinates, projections, and scale. Geographic coordinates for the nearly spherical world are measured in polar coordinates, angles of rotation in degrees, minutes, and seconds, or decimal degrees. The (0,0) origin is generally taken as the intersection of the equator with the prime meridian (great circle) passing through the poles and Greenwich, England. Longitude is measured to the east and west of the origin for up to 180° in each direction. Latitude is measured north and south for up to 90° in each direction.

The world is not quite a sphere because the poles are slightly flattened and the equator is slightly bulged out. The world's surface is better modeled by a spheroid, which has elliptical cross sections with two radii, instead of the one radius of a sphere. The mathematical representation of the world as a spheroid is called a datum; for example, two datums

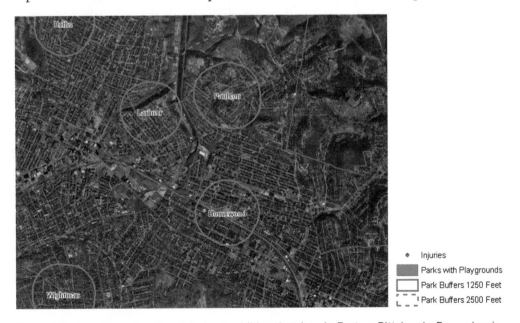

Legend:
- Injuries
- Parks with Playgrounds
- Park Buffers 1250 Feet
- Park Buffers 2500 Feet

Figure 1.2 Locations of serious injuries to child pedestrians in Eastern Pittsburgh, Pennsylvania.

Sources: (a) Children's Hospital of Pittsburg; (b) Pennsylvania Spatial Data Access (PASDA) and USGS; (c) City of Pittsburgh Department of City Planning.

commonly used for North America are NAD 1927 and NAD 1983. If you use the same projection, but with two different datums, then each corresponding map will have small but noticeable differences in coordinates.

A point, line, or polygon feature on the surface of the world is on a three-dimensional spheroid, whereas, features on a paper map or computer screen are on flat surfaces. The mathematical transformation of a world feature to a flat map is called a projection. There are many projections, some of which you will use in tutorial 4. Each projection has its own rectangular coordinate system with a (0,0) origin conveniently located so that coordinates generally are positive and have distance units, usually feet or meters.

Necessarily, all projections cause distortions of direction, shape, area, and length in some combination. So-called conformal projections preserve shape at the expense of distorting area. Some examples are the Mercator and Lambert conic projections. Equal area projections are the opposite of conformal projections: they preserve area while distorting shape. Examples are the cylindrical and Albers equal area projections (Clarke 2003, 42–44).

Map scale is often stated as a unitless, representative fraction; for example, 1:24,000 is a map scale where 1 inch on the map represents 24,000 inches on the ground, and any distance units can be substituted for inches. Small-scale maps have a vantage point far above the earth and large-scale maps are zoomed in to relatively small areas. Distortions are considerable for small-scale maps but negligible for large-scale maps relative to policy, planning, and research applications.

GIS maps are composites of overlaying map layers. For large-scale maps such as in figure 1.2, the bottom layer can be a raster map with one or more vector layers on top, placed in order so that smaller or more important features are on top and are not covered up by larger contextual features. Small-scale maps, such as figure 1.1, often consist of all vector map layers. Each vector layer consists of a homogeneous type of feature: points, lines, or polygons.

Digital map infrastructure

GIS is perhaps the only information technology that requires a major digital infrastructure: We also refer to the map layers of the infrastructure as basemaps, namely, a collection of standards, codes, and data designed, built, and maintained by government. Vendors provide valuable enhancements to the digital map infrastructure, but for the most part, it is a public good financed by tax dollars. Without this infrastructure, GIS would not be a viable technology.

The National Spatial Data Infrastructure (NSDI), developed by the Federal Geographic Data Committee (*www.fgdc.gov*), ". . . encompasses policies, standards, and procedures for organizations to cooperatively produce and share geographic data." Associated with the NSDI is the Geospatial One-Stop Web site (*gos2.geodata.gov*) for access to spatial data. Next we will briefly review several components of the NSDI.

Perhaps most useful for health applications are the TIGER/Line maps provided by the U.S. Census Bureau. These maps are available by states and counties for many classes of layers. These classes, and examples of each, follow:

+ *Political layers*—states, counties, county subdivisions (towns and cities), and voting districts
+ *Statistical layers*—census tracts, block groups, and blocks
+ *Administrative layers*—ZIP Codes and school districts
+ *Physical layers*—highways, streets, rivers, streams, lakes, and railroads

You can download TIGER/Line map layers in GIS-ready formats at no cost from a variety of Web sites, including the U.S. Census Bureau site (*www.census.gov*) and the ESRI site (*www.esri.com*). Steps for doing so are found in tutorial 5.

Corresponding to TIGER/Line maps of statistical boundaries is census data tabulated by census and federal information processing standards (FIPS) codes (*www.census.gov/geo/www /fips/fips.html*) and census-area codes. FIPS codes are ". . . a standardized set of numeric or alphabetic codes issued by the National Institute of Standards and Technology (NIST) to ensure uniform identification of geographic entities through all federal government agencies." Data from the decennial census is available at no cost from *www.census.gov/geo/www*. Steps for downloading census data and preparing it for GIS use with TIGER/Line maps are also found in tutorial 5.

The U.S. Geological Survey (see *www.usgs.gov/aboutusgs*) is the "largest water, earth, and biological science and civilian mapping agency . . . [and it] collects, monitors, analyzes, and provides scientific understanding about natural resource conditions, issues, and problems." Among its products useful for health applications are its 1:24,000-, 1:25,000-, 1:63,360-scale topographic maps, known as digital raster graphic (DRG) maps in scanned image format, and its digital orthophoto quarter quadrangle (DOQQ) aerial photographs (such as are used in figure 1.2). Full national coverage of the most recent DOQQs and 90 percent of DRG maps are available at nominal cost from the Seamless Data Distribution System at *edcsns17.cr.usgs .gov/EarthExplorer*.

Local governments provide many of the large-scale map layers in the United States, and in this data most features are smaller than a city block. Included are deeded land parcels and corresponding real property data files on land parcels, structures, owners, building roof footprints, and pavement digitized from aerial photographs. Often you can obtain such map layers and data for nominal prices from local governments.

Unique capabilities of GIS

Historically, maps were made for reference purposes. Examples of reference maps are street maps, atlases, and the USGS topographic maps. It wasn't until GIS, however, that analytic mapping became widely possible. For analytic mapping, an analyst collects and compiles map layers for the problem at hand, builds a database, and then uses GIS functionality to provide information for understanding or solving a problem. Before GIS, analytic mapping was limited to a few kinds of organizations, such as city planning departments. Analysts did not have digital map layers, so they made hard-copy drawings on acetate sheets that could be overlaid and switched in and out, for example, to show before-and-after maps for a new facility such as a baseball stadium. With GIS, however, anyone can easily add, subtract, turn on and off, and modify map layers in an analytic map composition. This capacity has led to a revolution in geography and an entirely new tool for organizations of all kinds.

As figures 1.1 and 1.2 show, maps use symbols that are defined in map legends. Graphical elements of symbols include fill color, pattern, and boundaries for polygons; width, color, and type (solid, dashed, etc.) for lines; and shape, color, and outline for points. A GIS analyst does not apply symbols individually to features, but applies and renders a layer at a time based on attribute values associated with geographic features.

For example, given a code attribute for schools with values public, private, and parochial, a GIS analyst can choose a green, circular, 10-point marker for public schools; a blue, square, 8-point marker for private schools; and an orange, triangular, 8-point marker for parochial schools. Those three steps render all schools in a map layer with desired point markers.

Similarly, we created the color-shaded county map layer in figure 1.1 based on an attribute that provides the lung cancer mortality rate of white males by county. A map that uses fill color in polygons for coding is called a choropleth map. In this case it shows an equal-interval numeric scale, rendered using a gray monochromatic color scale. The darker the shade of gray, the higher the interval of the numeric scale. By making selections and setting parameters, the GIS analyst accomplishes all of this coding and rendering with a simple graphical user interface.

Most organizations generate or collect data that includes street addresses, ZIP Codes, or other georeferences. GIS is able to spatially enable such data, that is, add geographic coordinates or make data records joinable to boundary maps. Geocoding, also known as address matching, uses street addresses as input and assigns point coordinates to address records on or adjacent to street centerlines, such as in the TIGER/Line street maps. Geocoding uses a sophisticated program with built-in intelligence—similar to a postal delivery person's when delivering your mail—that can interpret misspellings, variations in abbreviations, and so on.

Policy, planning, and research activities often require data aggregated over space and time, rather than individual points. For example, in a study of demand patterns for locating a satellite medical clinic, it may be desirable to aggregate patient residence data to counts per census tract or ZIP Code boundaries for a recent year. GIS has the unique capacity to determine the areas in which points lie, using a spatial join or overlay function, and this enables the analyst to count points or summarize their attributes (e.g., using sums or averages) by area.

This brings us to the last GIS capability to be described in this section: proximity analysis. As an example, we conducted a study to determine whether the decline in the use of senior centers was affected by the distance from the seniors' residences (Johnson, et al. 2005). We geocoded the senior centers that provided human services and where the senior citizens lived, placing them as points on a map, and included the total target population using census data by city block. Then we used ArcGIS to create buffers around the facilities with a radius of 0.5 miles, 1 mile, 1.5 miles, 2.0 miles, and so on. We used spatial joins to assign buffer identifiers to residence points and blocks, count clients by buffer area, and sum population by block group.

Next, through careful subtraction of counts and sums, we were able to get the total number of clients and the target population in each ring around facilities (e.g., 0.5 miles, 1 mile, 1.5 miles), calculate use rates for each ring by dividing the count of clients by the sum of target population, and plot the relationship of use rate versus mean distance of each ring from facilities. We found that the use rate by the clients, who were elderly users of the senior center facilities in our county, declined rapidly with distance, given their mobility limitations. The policy implication of this result is that senior centers need to be located in areas with high densities of elderly populations. You will conduct similar buffer analyses in tutorials 7, 9, and 10 in a variety of health contexts.

Tutorial 1: Introducing GIS and health applications

Health care is a large, growing, and complex sector of economies around the world. The United States, like other countries, faces many challenges in providing the best health care for its citizens and at the lowest possible cost. Currently many health informatics systems are manual and/or nonintegrated (*The Economist* 2005). By nonintegrated, we mean that interacting organizations have information systems in-house that are not connected with each other in ways that allow sharing of data that could be beneficial. This has led to top-heavy administrations, high costs of transactions (Hagland 2004), medical errors, and duplication of efforts, such as unnecessary medical tests (Protti 2005). Additional health-policy issues arise, for example, from too much emphasis on treatment of sickness and not enough on prevention of illness (Kennedy 2004); enormous numbers of uninsured persons; the overuse of emergency rooms; nursing shortages; and lack of preparedness for bioterrorism (Featherly 2004).

One clear trend in health policy, research, planning, and management is the increasingly important role of health informatics. More systems will become automated and integrated, with large costs but even larger benefits. What does this mean for GIS applications? One consequence is that there will be even more data available for possible input to GIS—additional data on patients, facilities, programs, and events that include disease incidence, medical diagnostics, and treatments. Much of the additional data will have street addresses, ZIP Codes, or other location elements that will make them applicable to GIS processing.

This book has a sampling of health GIS applications that cut a wide path across the landscape we have just described. Next is a brief summary of the tutorials ahead.

Tutorial 2: Visualizing health data

First is a simple public health application for visualizing breast cancer mortality rates at the state and county levels across the United States. In the tutorial, you will work with breast cancer data and lung cancer data. While valuable for providing a snapshot of cancer mortality, the primary purpose of the application is to get you comfortable with map navigation in ArcGIS. ArcGIS provides many ways to change scales and views of a map in search of information, as well as ways to work with the data records behind the map features. You will get experience with some of them in this tutorial.

Tutorial 3: Designing maps for a health study

In tutorial 3 we will learn about uninsured populations in a state and their health-care financial needs. In the tutorial, you will analyze where to locate programs that provide health-related financial support for uninsured populations in Texas counties. You will use an advanced map with a bivariate analysis to contrast the magnitude of uninsured populations with measures of poverty by county.

GIS can provide many kinds of outputs. In this tutorial you will build stand-alone map layouts, with components such as multiple map frames, legends, and scale bars to use in presentations and reports. In the exercises you will use U.S. Census data to explore neighborhoods for areas in which to promote walking for reducing obesity.

Tutorial 4: Projecting and using spatial data

What are the most appropriate ways to map disease incidence (numbers of cases) versus prevalence (numbers of cases per population of 10,000). In the first health application you will visualize a communicable disease, HIV infection, and AIDS. You will build two kinds of map layers, one for disease incidence based on polygon centroids (points) using size-graduated point markers and the other for disease prevalence represented by fill color for polygons to encode data.

A second application further pursues the problem of child obesity. Here your objective will be to identify green spaces in the vicinity of schools for possible use in physical education programs.

GIS issues pursued for these applications involve importing spatial data into ArcGIS and projecting map layers for the application and geographic scale at hand. The exercises in this tutorial address the same GIS issues, but move into an entirely new application area—preparation of emergency evacuation routes to medical facilities and shelters.

Tutorial 5: Downloading and preparing spatial data

Where are the concentrations of a city's older houses that are likely to have lead-based paint? Do children who have elevated levels of lead in their blood live in those areas? The purpose of this study is to identify clusters of children with elevated levels for targeting screening programs. You will work with blood samples and census data on housing built before 1970, when lead-based paints were still used.

In this tutorial you will download and prepare U.S. Census data. You must clean up the data by renaming variables and deleting rows that do not conform to data table formats, modifying census tract identifiers in the table so that they match comparable identifiers in the census tract map layer, and joining them to a downloaded census tract boundary map. Ultimately, you will produce a very nice bivariate map using choropleth and dot density displays. In that map, you will place randomly located points within polygons in proportion to an attribute of interest. The exercises in this tutorial seek additional explanation of observed clusters by using additional census variables.

Tutorial 6: Geocoding tabular data

General spatial information is available from basemaps, but how do you get your organization's data for points on a map? Data of interest often includes point locations of patients' or clients' residences, health care or other service delivery locations, such as the scenes of traffic accidents. If data includes street addresses, ZIP Codes, or other spatial identifiers, then GIS has the tools to plot points of interest to use for analysis.

For this case study, you need to spatially enable some data currently in tabular form. You will geocode existing facilities within a county so they can be placed on a map as points. You also will place patients on a ZIP Code map over a wide area. With this data mapped, you can readily see potential service gaps. Then, in an exercise, you will map some suitability measures for a health clinic location, to aid in identifying locations in gap areas that would be an attractive site for a new facility.

Tutorial 7: Preparing and analyzing spatial data

What are some neighborhood factors leading to child pedestrian injuries in a city? Is poverty a factor? What about the lack of safe public areas for play? In this tutorial you will explore the determinants of serious child pedestrian injuries for the purpose of designing prevention programs. The basis of your study is a sample of serious injury data that has been geocoded and can be compared to census data on poverty and map layers for streets, neighborhoods, and parks that have playgrounds and playing fields.

The GIS work includes preparatory steps for extracting study-region maps from county maps and then focuses on detailed proximity analyses using park buffers, like those seen in figure 1.2.

Tutorial 8: Transforming data using approximate methods

How can health-care analysts combine data from different, incompatible polygon boundary sets? Often the spatial unit of analysis for a health study will be a custom set of polygon boundaries, designed for the phenomenon at hand. An example is the hospital service areas and hospital referral regions of the Dartmouth Atlas of Health Care Project of the Center for the Evaluative Clinical Sciences at Dartmouth Medical School (*www.dartmouthatlas.org*) in Hanover, New Hampshire. While appropriate for studying patterns in the quality of health care across the country, these custom areas have the limitation of not sharing boundaries with census statistical areas (i.e., they are noncoterminous sets of boundaries). Thus, it is not possible to directly use census data for supportive analysis of the custom areas.

Another common case is regional analysis in which individual records have only ZIP Codes as spatial identifiers, so ZIP Codes become the *de facto* unit of spatial analysis. Detailed census variables, from U.S. Census Summary File 3 on income, poverty, educational employment, and so on, are not easily available at the ZIP Code level. Fortunately, advanced GIS functionality, using spatial joins, can produce some very accurate approximations (i.e., apportionments) for transforming data from one set of polygons to another incompatible set.

Tutorial 9: Using ArcGIS Spatial Analyst for demand estimation

This tutorial is an introduction to the Spatial Analyst extension for ArcGIS Desktop. Spatial Analyst uses or creates raster datasets comprised of grid cells to display data that is distributed continuously over space as a surface. In this tutorial you will prepare and analyze a demand surface map for the location of heart defibrillators in Pittsburgh, with demand based on the number of out-of-hospital cardiac arrests with potential bystander help. You will also learn how to use Spatial Analyst's raster calculator to create a poverty index surface combined with several census data measures from block and block group polygon layers.

Tutorial 10: Case study: Studying food-borne disease outbreaks

Finally, this tutorial and tutorial 11 provide a change of pace—opportunities to apply and extend the GIS skills and health applications you have learned in the previous nine tutorials to new case studies. We provide source data and guidelines for analysis, with a broad outline of steps; however, it is up to you to carry out the GIS work somewhat independently. In this tutorial, you will prepare map layers, which includes geocoding, as the basis for analyzing outbreaks of food-borne illnesses. Then you will use data to simulate the impact of an outbreak. You will do a proximity analysis based on patterns in reported disease cases.

Tutorial 11: Case study: Forming a national ACHE chapter

The book concludes with a second case study, following a similar setup to that in tutorial 10. Staff members of the American College of Healthcare Executives (ACHE) want you to use GIS to help them set up ACHE chapters across the country that provide educational and other services to health-care professionals.

You will perform a buffer analysis of existing affiliates that propose to become ACHE chapters. The buffers will help determine territories served and gaps that suggest where new chapters should be established. You will do some work interactively using ArcGIS, but then for steps that must be done repeatedly over time, you will build an ArcGIS model that generates a macro to automate steps.

Introduction to ArcGIS and map documents

ArcGIS Desktop is available in three license levels: ArcView, ArcEditor, and ArcInfo. All three of the licensed ArcGIS Desktop products look and work the same, though they differ in how much they can do.

This book is designed for use with ArcGIS Desktop 9.3 software with an ArcView license. ArcView, the most popular member of this collection and most widely used GIS package in the world, is a full-featured GIS software application for visualizing, managing, creating, and analyzing geographic data. ArcEditor adds more GIS editing tools to ArcView. ArcInfo is the most comprehensive GIS package, adding advanced data conversion and geoprocessing capabilities to ArcEditor. While this book was written for ArcView, you can use it with ArcEditor and ArcInfo as well.

Also available as part of ArcGIS is the free ArcReader mapping application, which allows users to view, explore, and print maps. Finally, ArcGIS has numerous extensions that can be added to ArcView, ArcEditor, and ArcInfo. Some major extensions include ArcGIS 3D Analyst for three-dimensional rendering of surfaces, ArcGIS Network Analyst for routing and other street network applications, and ArcGIS Spatial Analyst for generating and working with raster maps.

ArcView consists of two application programs, ArcCatalog and ArcMap. ArcCatalog is a utility program that has file browsing, data importing and converting, and file maintenance functions (such as create, copy, and delete)—all with special features for GIS source data. For managing GIS source data, you will use ArcCatalog instead of the Microsoft Windows utilities My Computer or Windows Explorer.

GIS analysts use ArcMap to compose a map from basemap layers, and then they can carry out many kinds of analyses and produce several GIS outputs. A map composition is saved in a map document file with a name chosen by the user and the .mxd file extension. For example, you will soon open Tutorial1A.mxd.

A map document stores pointers (paths) to map layers, data tables, and other data sources for use in a map composition, but does not store a copy of any data source. Consequently, map layers can be stored anywhere on your computer, local area network, or even on an Internet server, and be part of your map document. In this book, you will use data sources available from the data CD accompanying the book that you will install on your desktop computer's hard drive.

Installing ArcView and the health tutorial data CD

This book includes a DVD with the 180-day trial version of ArcGIS Desktop 9.3. See appendix C for instructions on installing ArcView and the data CD, also accompanying the book. You must successfully install ArcView and the data to complete the tutorials in this book.

Introducing the ArcGIS user interface

The following steps will acquaint you with the functionality and user interfaces of ArcMap and ArcCatalog. You will start by using ArcCatalog to browse the data sources used in figure 1.1 (see p. 2), and then examine the completed project itself. You will learn how to build, modify, and query data in the remaining tutorials.

In the exercises that follow, you need to be at your computer to carry out the numbered steps. Screen captures accompanying the steps show you important dialog boxes and output. Occasionally we have added "Your Turn" exercises after a series of steps. It's critical that you do these brief exercises to start internalizing the processes covered.

Launch ArcCatalog

1   **From the Windows taskbar, click Start, All Programs, ArcGIS, ArcCatalog.**

Depending on how ArcGIS has been installed, you may have a different navigation menu or a name other than ArcGIS.

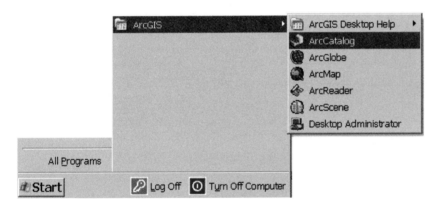

2   **The left panel of ArcCatalog is called the Catalog tree. It is used to navigate to the data on your computer or network server, much like Windows Explorer. In the Catalog tree, navigate to your GistutorialHealth folder by clicking the small plus signs to expand the folders in which it's installed. (The default location for this folder is C:\GistutorialHealth, but it may be in a different location depending on where you or your instructor installed it. If you cannot find this folder, make sure it was installed as described in appendix B.) After navigating to the GistutorialHealth folder, expand the United States folder located inside it.**

The right panel, called the Catalog display, contains three tabs: Contents, Preview, and Metadata. When you choose the Contents tab, the datasets in the current folder are listed. The datasets currently listed represent spatial data, and the icon next to each file name indicates what type of geometry the data is built with: point, line, or polygon.

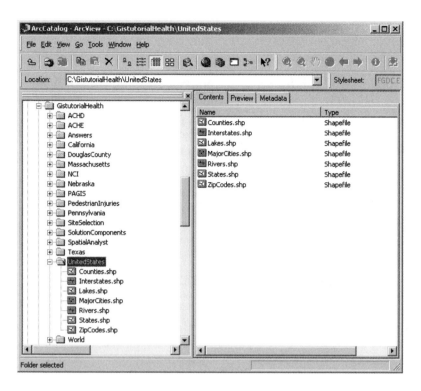

3 In the Catalog display, click States.shp, then click the Preview tab at the top of the right panel.

Previewing data this way allows you to get a quick glimpse of the data without actually loading it into a map. You can also use this tab to preview the contents of a table.

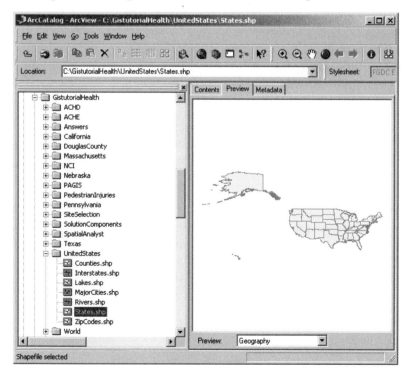

4   At the bottom of the Catalog display, click the Preview drop-down arrow and click Table, then use
     the horizontal scroll bar to view the attribute fields in the table.

Each record in the table corresponds to one of the state polygons you previewed in the previous step, and as you can see, there are quite a few attributes stored for each state, most of which are demographic. For example, by reading across the table, you could identify that the state of Washington is in the Pacific subregion and had a population of 5,894,121 in 2000. We used the STATE_NAME attribute to label states in figure 1.1.

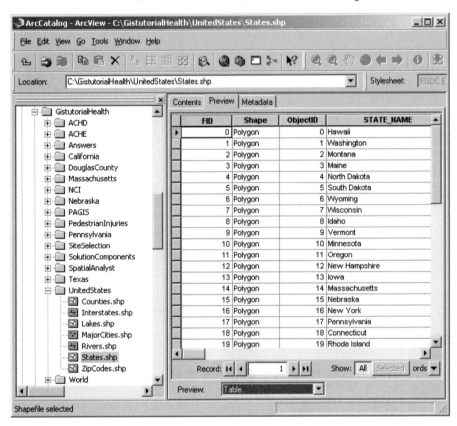

5   Click the Metadata tab at the top of the Catalog display and click the Spatial tab in the resulting
     display. (If the Spatial tab does not display, make sure the Stylesheet drop-down list is set to
     FGDC ESRI.)

Metadata describes data; it is data about data. For example, you can see that States has a geographic coordinate system (latitude and longitude) with certain bounding coordinates for the rectangle framing the map layer. Also available are descriptions of the data and a list of attributes with their data types, under the Description and Attributes buttons.

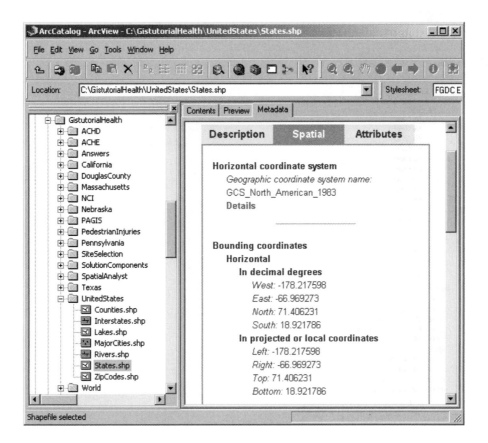

6   **Click the Contents tab in the Catalog display.**

YOUR TURN

Explore additional layers in the United States folder. When finished, click the contractor button with the minus sign to the left of the United States folder icon in the Catalog tree. Then close ArcCatalog.

Review data source types

You will do most GIS file maintenance work in ArcCatalog, though it is instructive to view GIS files in a conventional browser. Next you will examine two common ESRI file formats used in GIS: a shapefile and a personal geodatabase. A shapefile map layer has three or more files with the same name but different file extensions, all stored in the same folder. A personal geodatabase is a Microsoft Access database file (.mdb extension) that has one or more map layers stored as relational database tables. Both of these data types are very common in the GIS industry, with the geodatabase being a more modern form.

1   **From the Windows taskbar, click Start, My Computer. (The path to My Computer may differ depending on which operating system you are using.)**

2   Browse to where your **GistutorialHealth** folder is installed (e.g., C:\GistutorialHeath).

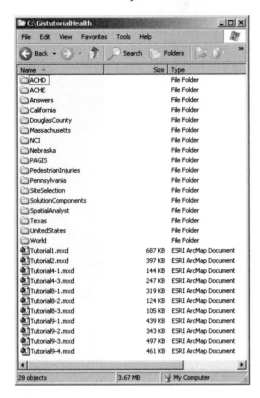

3   Double-click the United States folder to view its shapefiles.

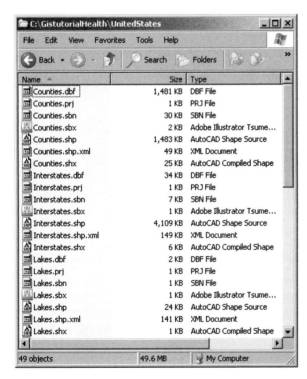

Let's review the MajorCities shapefile, which actually consists of seven files, all with the name MajorCities.

- The MajorCities file with the .shp extension has the features' geometry and coordinates. In this case, each record has a point and an x,y location. For line and polygon layers, each shape record has coordinates of a line segment or a polygon.
- The MajorCities file with the .dbf extension has the feature attribute table in dBASE format. This file can be opened and edited as a Microsoft Excel spreadsheet and an Access database, but such work must be done carefully and without deleting or adding records or changing the order of rows. This could result in corrupted data. The relationship between the .shp and .dbf files of a shapefile depends on one-to-one physical arrangement of records in both files.
- The .sbx and .shx files contain indexes for speeding up searches and queries. The .prj file is a simple text file that has the map projection parameters of the layer.
- Finally, the .shp.xml file has the layer's metadata and can be opened in a Web browser for reading.

4   Click View, Go To, Up One Level in My Computer.

5   Click the Solution Components folder icon, then click the Chapter 5 folder.

This folder contains a personal geodatabase, LeadStudy.mdb. A single personal geodatabase can have one or more vector map layers and data tables. Never open a personal geodatabase in Microsoft Access! Always use ArcCatalog to maintain map layers and data tables stored in a personal geodatabase; otherwise, you will likely corrupt the layers.

6   Close My Computer.

YOUR TURN

Launch ArcCatalog and explore the personal geodatabase in the **\GistutorialHealth \SolutionsComponents\Chapter5** folder. Preview its tables and map layer. Then close ArcCatalog.

Launch ArcMap

1 From the Windows taskbar, click Start, All Programs, ArcGIS, ArcMap.

Depending on how ArcGIS and ArcMap have been installed, you may have a different navigation menu or a name other than ArcGIS.

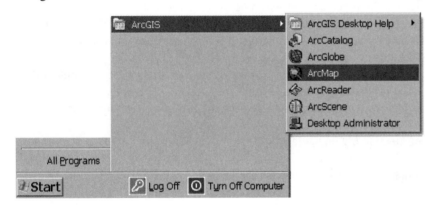

2 In the resulting ArcMap window, click the An existing map radio button, then click OK.

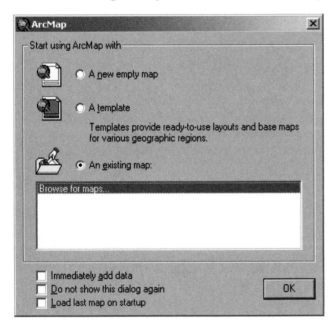

3 Browse to the drive and folder in which the **GistutorialHealth** folder is installed (e.g., **C:\GistutorialHealth**).

4   Click the **Tutorial1.mxd** map document icon, then click Open.

Note: The .mxd extensions may not be visible, depending on how your operating system is configured.

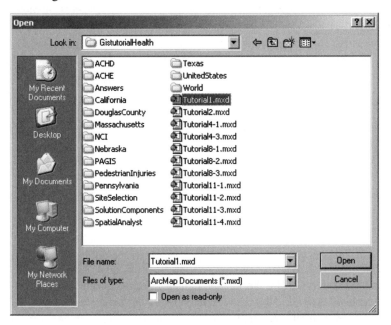

Tutorial1.mxd opens in the ArcMap application window. If you do not see the table of contents, click View, Table of Contents to add this panel. The map currently contains the contiguous United States showing demographics related to female-headed households and lung cancer mortality rates. The major components of the ArcMap interface are also identified.

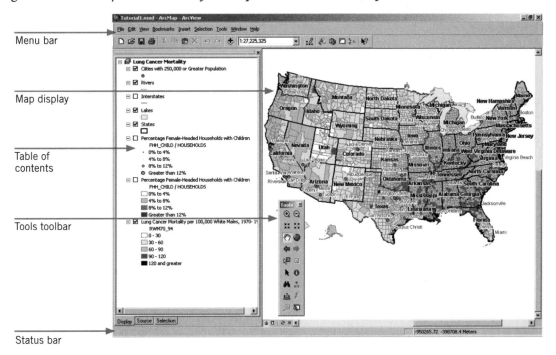

Let's review the major components of the ArcMap application window.

- The map display is where the datasets loaded into the map are drawn.
- The table of contents lists all the data in the map document and allows you to toggle their visibility and access their properties. Currently, the Display tab is selected at the bottom of the table of contents showing the order of map layers and their legends. By clicking the Source tab at the bottom of the table of contents, you can also see the folder and file path to the source data of map layers and tables. ArcMap draws maps from the bottom up in the table of contents, so big feature layers, such as Lung Cancer Mortality, that would cover smaller feature layers, such as Rivers, must go on the bottom. You can see that only some of the layers are turned on, those with checked boxes.
- The Tools toolbar has frequently used tools and can be docked, if desired, by dragging it by its blue top to any boundary in the ArcMap interface. Similarly, you can undock it by dragging and dropping it to the desired location.
- The menu bar has some items common to most Windows application packages, plus some unique to GIS.
- The status bar displays the map coordinates of the cursor location in the map display. In the graphic on the previous page, the cursor is currently over Omaha, Nebraska, and the coordinates for Omaha are being displayed on the status bar.

YOUR TURN

Experiment with turning map layers on and off by checking and unchecking the boxes to the left of each map layer in the table of contents. Start with layers currently turned off, from the top down, and turn each one on and then off. Then try various combinations. Keep in mind that the Female-Headed Households with Children layer is a strong indicator of poverty. Of course, not every such household is in poverty, but the tendency is strong. When finished, return the map document to its original condition, with layers turned on and off as seen on the previous page.

View map layer attribute tables

1   In the table of contents, right-click Cities with 250,000 or Greater Population. Select Open
    Attribute Table.

Attributes of Cities with 250,000 or Greater Population opens. This is the same sort of table
that you previewed in ArcCatalog.

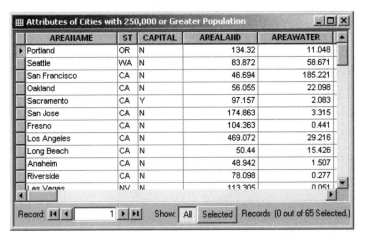

2   Visually scan the map for a few cities listed in the table, verifying that there is a point plotted for
    every record in the table.

3   Close the table.

TURN

YOUR

Open a few other tables and scan the contents.

View map layer properties

1   In the table of contents, right-click **Cities with 250,000 or Greater Population** and in the resulting context menu, click **Properties**. In the resulting **Layer Properties** dialog box, click the **General** tab.

The Layer Properties is an important dialog box for managing the way layers behave and appear in ArcMap. We will not attempt to describe all the properties that can be set, but will just review useful ones to know about for now. For example, on this panel of the Layer Properties you can change the layer name by typing the name of your choice into the Layer Name text box.

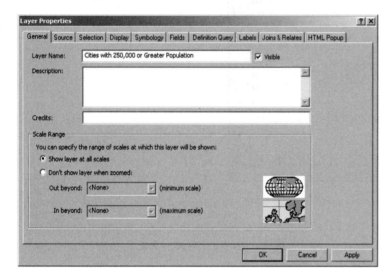

2   In the Layer Properties dialog box, click the **Source** tab.

This window provides bounding coordinates of the map layer (i.e., its extent), the data type, location on the server or computer, geometry type, and projection.

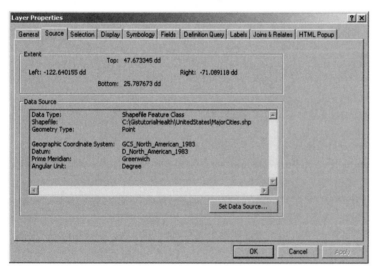

3   **Click the Symbology tab.**

This tab provides many options for symbolizing vector map layers. The cities layer uses a single symbol, a purple circular point marker with a black outline, chosen by the authors.

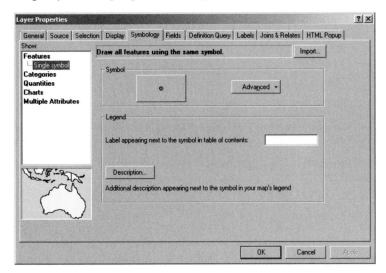

4   **Click the Fields tab.**

This tab lists the layer's attribute fields and their properties.

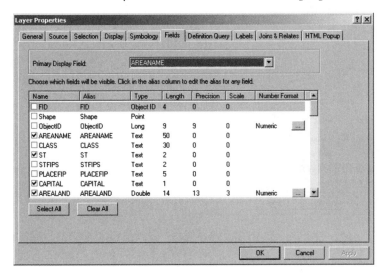

5   **Click the Definition Query tab.**

Use this tab to restrict what is displayed within a map layer. In this case, we used the POP2000 attribute to limit cities displayed to those with a population of 250,000 or more in the year 2000. This only changes the display and does not remove the records from the source data.

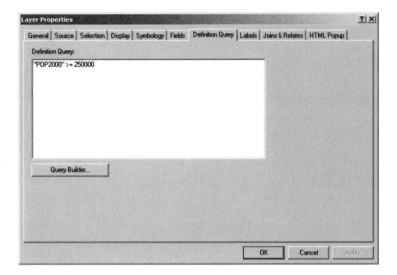

6 Click the Labels tab.

This tab allows you to label features, if you wish, using an attribute from the feature attribute table. We used AREANAME, which is the name of cities, with a purple font and white halo mask. We also turned labeling on with the check box at the top of the form.

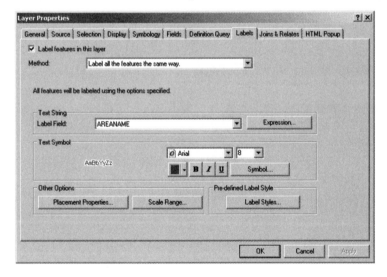

7 Close Layer Properties.

YOUR TURN

Examine the properties of a few more layers, but do not make any changes. When finished, close ArcMap.

Use the map

Fundamentally, when you use GIS for analysis, you observe spatial patterns related to a problem, phenomenon, or issue of interest. In this case, the phenomenon is mortality of white males from lung cancer.

Clearly we can see strong spatial patterns with concentrations of mortality along the southeastern coast of the United States and other locations. We can recognize some correlates on the map, based on spatial arrangement alone. For example, the band of high mortality along the eastern border of Kentucky is in that state's coal mining belt. Perhaps the white males succumbing to lung cancer in that area tend to be coal miners.

Some of the southeastern peak areas for mortality correspond to tobacco-growing areas of Virginia, the Carolinas, and Georgia, but high mortality areas run beyond the tobacco fields. Perhaps being near to tobacco-growing areas increases the likelihood of smoking and, therefore, lung cancer. A question then becomes: how far beyond the immediate tobacco growing areas could such an influence exist? Regardless, it cannot account for the high mortality observed along the Mississippi River.

An additional correlation is poverty, which contributes to many health problems and perhaps increases exposure to factors leading to lung cancer. A strong indicator of poverty, and the only poverty indicator available in our U.S. counties data, is the percentage of female-headed households with children. As an example of this indicator's effectiveness, in Pittsburgh at the tract level the simple correlation between percentage of female-headed households with children and percentage of total population below the poverty line is 0.67. Let's see if there is any visual evidence of a positive correlation of this poverty indicator with white male lung cancer incidence.

As you will see, we have used a size-graduated point marker and dichromatic color scale for this poverty indicator. We used an equal-interval numeric scale of 4 percent width, with the darker shade of green signifying the lowest value interval and the darker shade of orange signifying the highest value interval. Also, the larger the diameter of circular point marker used, the higher the interval of the indicator variable.

1   **Open ArcMap and open Tutorial1.mxd. Check the box to the left of the Percentage Female-Headed Households with Children map layer in the table of contents to turn that layer on.**

Immediately, you can see that this variable is promising as a correlation to the male lung cancer deaths because it is high in many of the same areas where lung cancer mortality is high. The current map scale, however, is zoomed out too far. You need a closer look at the southeastern United States. We have built a spatial bookmark for this purpose, which you will use next, to get an uncluttered, zoomed-in view of the map. Notice that the map scale in the graphic on the following page is 1:27,183,632 for the entire United States. It will be different on your screen, because your screen is likely a different physical size than ours. Make a note of your scale.

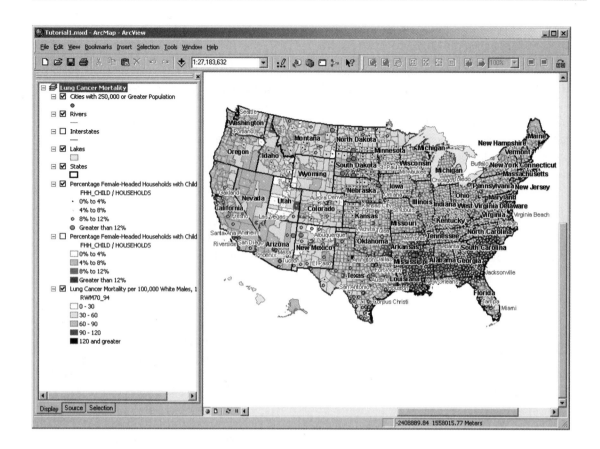

2   **From the Bookmarks menu, click SouthEast.**

That helped considerably. You can see that there is a visual correlation, with both variables tending to be high in the same areas. Clearly, further examination would require a multivariate model. We have identified some promising variables: coal production, tobacco crops, adjacency to tobacco-growing areas, and poverty. For the present, however, you need a professional-quality map that could be used in a Microsoft Office Word document or PowerPoint presentation. We have built a map layout for this purpose, which you will view next. Note that the map scale is much larger when zoomed in to 1:11,372,806, as shown in the following graphic.

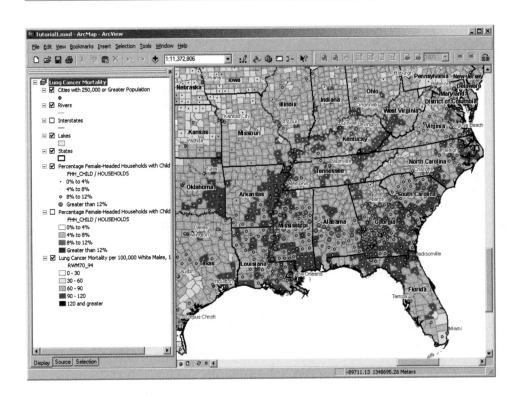

3   From the View menu, click Layout View.

Below is the resultant map, which you will later learn how to export for use in a document. ArcMap provides two general views: data view and layout view. Typically you use data view to interact with your map data through browsing, symbolizing, and editing. You can also interact with your data in layout view, but its primary purpose is to finalize map compositions. In layout view you can add north arrows, scale bars, legends, and other map elements.

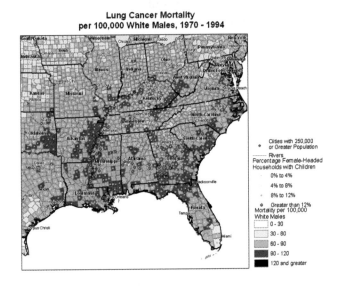

4   From the Bookmarks menu, click U.S.

5   Close ArcMap. Do not save your changes.

Summary

GIS is a fascinating and valuable information technology, enabling spatial processing and visualization of data in ways never before possible. At the most basic level, GIS makes it easy to quickly compose and render maps from base layers. You can easily turn map layers on and off to study spatial patterns and correlations. You saw how GIS connects visual maps and underlying attribute data when you labeled map features and rendered numeric scales for variables using choropleth and graduated point marker maps. In later tutorials, you will discover additional, powerful uses for attribute data connected to map features.

Two components make GIS analysis possible for applications such as in health care. The first is the national map infrastructure—a collection of basemaps, census and other data, and geocodes for uniquely identifying areas. In the United States, this resource is a public good, paid for by tax dollars, and available for your use at no or nominal cost. Commercial map layers are also available at reasonable cost, and in many cases are essential for applications. This tutorial introduced important components of map layers, including geographic and rectangular coordinate systems, projections between the two types of coordinate systems, and map scale.

The second component necessary for applications is user-friendly and powerful GIS software. ArcGIS Desktop is the world's leading GIS software and the software used in this book. This tutorial covers the primary uses and interfaces of the two major ArcGIS application packages: the ArcCatalog utility for browsing and maintaining spatial data files, and ArcMap for creating maps and analyzing data. This tutorial asks you to examine the input map layers and GIS data for studying lung cancer mortality in white males. The spatial patterns you observed suggest some possible correlations of the mortality data, including poverty, tobacco growing, and coal mining.

We should probably add a third necessary component for successful GIS applications: GIS analysts. There is a lot to learn, and knowing how to use GIS is not a common skill. Nevertheless, this book will help you use GIS productively and efficiently, making the best use of your limited and valuable time.

References

Clarke, K. C. 2003. *Getting started with geographic information systems.* 4th ed. Upper Saddle River: Prentice Hall.

Featherly, K. 2004. Battling bioterror. Healthcare informatics online. www.healthcare-informatics. com/issues/2004/02_04/cover.htm#disease (no longer available).

Hagland, M. 2004. Harnessing efficiency. *Healthcare informatics online.* www.healthcare-informatics. com/issues/2004/02_04/cover.htm#workflow (no longer available).

Johnson, M., W. L. Gorr, and S. Roehrig. 2005. Location of service facilities for the elderly. *Annals of operations research* 136:1.

Kennedy, E. May 13, 2004. Statement on the introduction of the health care modernization, cost reduction, and quality improvement act. kennedy.senate.gov/~kennedy/ statements/04/05/2004513C28.html (no longer available).

Protti, D. J. 2005. The use of computers in health care can reduce errors, improve patient safety, and enhance the quality of service-there is evidence. www.connectingforhealth.nhs.uk/worldview/ protti2.

The Economist. 2005. Special report: IT in the health-care industry. April 30, 2005, 65.

Exercise assignment 1-1

Benchmark health GIS Web sites

Problem:

Many health organizations make maps available online. Examples include the World Health Organization at *www.who.int/csr/mapping/en*, the Centers for Disease Control at *www.cdc.gov/nchs/gis.htm*, and the National Cancer Institute at *www3.cancer.gov/atlasplus*. Note: Some URLs may change. If you cannot access the sites for the World Health Organization, Centers for Disease Control, or National Cancer Institute, try to find similar sites. The objective of this assignment is to investigate the unique capabilities of GIS and its applications to health by exploring these sites. Start by studying the above Web sites. Then browse the Internet to find an interesting health-related Web site that uses GIS (excluding the sites already listed above).

Provide an analysis of the Web site in a Microsoft PowerPoint presentation. Include the following in your presentation:

- Title page with title, Web site URL, and your name
- Purpose of the Web site and its use of GIS
- Screen captures of the Web site (about half a dozen) with maps
- A brief analysis of the GIS that includes:
  – GIS content provided
  – GIS functionality provided
  – Effectiveness in providing information
  – Ease of use
- Summary of what makes the Web site valuable in terms of functionality and content

What to turn in:

If you are working in a classroom setting with an instructor, you may be required to submit the PowerPoint slides that you created in the exercise.

PowerPoint slide

C:\GistutorialHealth\Answers\Assignment1\Assignment1.ppt

OBJECTIVES

Visualize breast cancer mortality by county across the United States
Understand how a GIS map is made up of map layers
Learn how to navigate a map using zooming, panning, and bookmarks
Understand and use the connection between visual map features and
tabular data
Learn how to select subsets of map features for processing
Learn how to find map features
Use data sorting records and labeling features to produce information

GIS Tutorial 2

Visualizing health data

Health-care scenario

According to the National Cancer Society, breast cancer remains the most frequently diagnosed cancer in women in the United States. Determining top geographic areas where breast cancer deaths occur may lead health officials to provide better targeted screening or interventions.

Solution approach

You are just starting to use ArcGIS, so this tutorial necessarily focuses on the basics of understanding and using GIS. To begin, you will work with an existing GIS document that you will open in ArcMap and modify by adding and symbolizing a map layer. With the map document in usable form, you will explore the map and associated attribute data using several GIS tools:

* Zoom, pan, and set spatial bookmarks for getting close-up views of the map in selected areas of the U.S.
* Find and identify for finding features and accessing their attribute data for reading
* Select to work with subsets of map layers; sort records for identifying top cancer counties
* Label and annotate to add information to maps

Your final output in this tutorial will be a map of the state of Texas highlighting the top five counties in terms of breast cancer mortality, with major cities displayed as points.

Manipulate map layers in a map document

In the first part of this tutorial you will learn the basics of the ArcMap software package. You will begin by opening an existing map document and learning how to add and manipulate map layers.

Launch ArcMap and open an existing map document

1 **From the Windows taskbar, click Start, All Programs, ArcGIS, ArcMap.**

Depending on how ArcGIS and ArcMap have been installed, you may have a different navigation menu or a name other than ArcGIS.

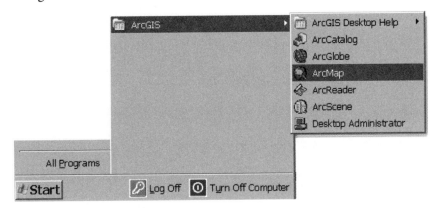

2 **In the resulting ArcMap window, click the An existing map radio button, then click OK.**

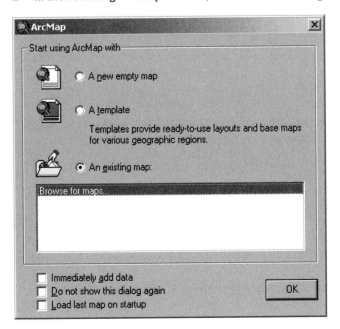

3   Browse to the drive and folder where you installed the **GistutorialHealth** folder
    (e.g., **C:\GistutorialHealth**).

4   Click the **Tutorial2.mxd** (or **Tutorial2**) map document icon, and click Open.

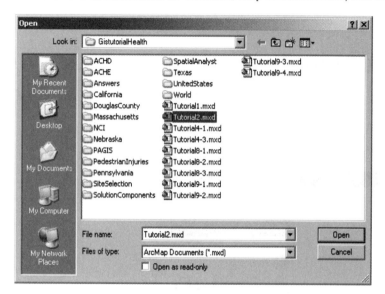

The resultant map of U.S. cities and states has two map layers already included and symbolized. The first layer is Major U.S. Cities (with population over 100,000). The second layer is Breast Cancer Deaths by State 1990-1994. We downloaded this data from the National Cancer Institute's cancer mortality maps and graphs Web site, *www3.cancer.gov/atlasplus*.

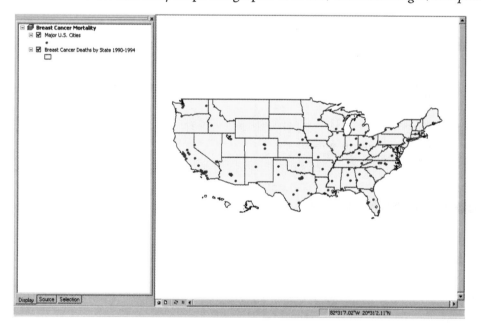

Add a layer

You can add more map layers to your map for more detailed analysis. For example, the National Cancer Institute collects data by county as well as by state. You can add a layer of data showing breast cancer mortality rates and number of deaths per county from 1970 to 1994. This data was saved as an ArcView shapefile, which contains the polygon features for counties and related data on death rates.

1   **Click the Add Data button.**

2   **In the Add Data dialog box, browse to \GistutorialHealth\NCI.**

3   **Click the BreCounty_7094.shp layer.**

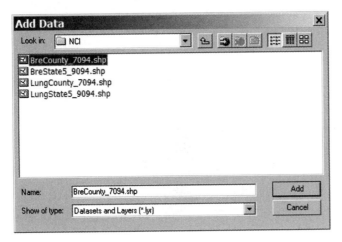

4   **Click Add.**

ArcMap chooses a random color for the counties layer. You can change the color later.

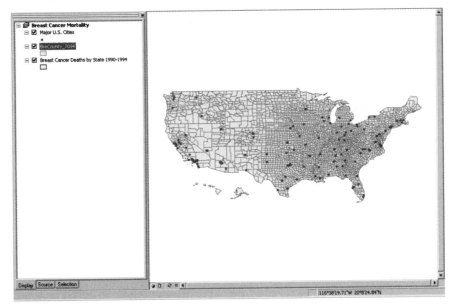

Change a layer's display order

Changing a layer's display order is important because features may be covered up by other features in your map. ArcView draws map layers from the bottom up, so if larger features are on top of smaller features, the smaller ones will not display.

1   **Click and hold down the left mouse button on the Major U.S. Cities layer.**

2   **Drag the Major U.S. Cities layer to the bottom of the table of contents and release.**

Because the cities layer is now drawn first, its points are covered by the states and counties layers and cannot be seen.

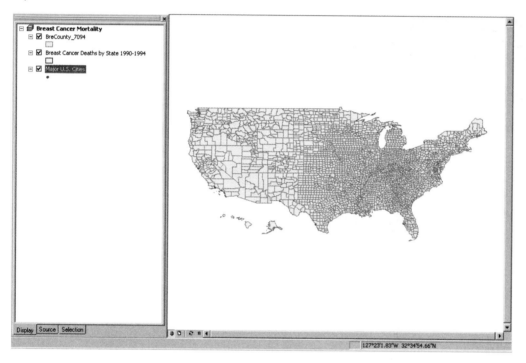

3   **Click and hold down the left mouse button on the Major U.S. Cities layer.**

4   **Drag the Major U.S. Cities layer back to the top of the table of contents and release.**

Because the cities layer is now drawn last, its points can be seen again.

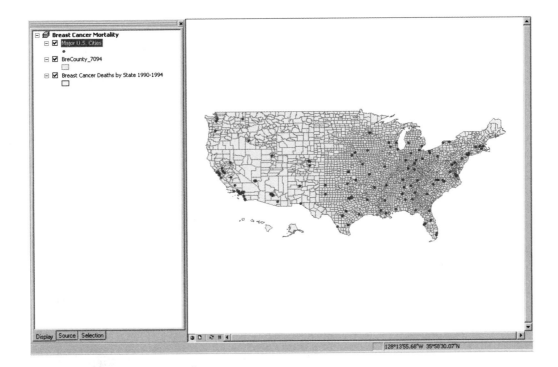

Drag the BreCounty_7094 layer to the bottom of the list and observe what happens. Then drag it back to the middle of the three layers.

Rename a layer

You will notice that when you initially add a layer, ArcMap uses the name of the shapefile as the default name of the layer in the table of contents. You will often want to change the name of the layer to a label that is easier to understand.

1   **In the table of contents, right-click the BreCounty_7094 layer.**

2   **Click Properties.**

3   **Click the General tab and change the layer name to Breast Cancer Deaths by County 1970-1994.**

4   **Click OK.**

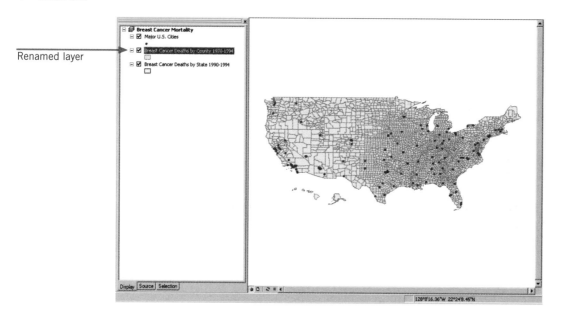

Renamed layer

Change a boundary layer's fill color

To better see the U.S. counties, you will want to change the color properties of both the county and state layers. First, you will change the counties to a white fill color with a light gray outline.

1   **In the table of contents, click the layer symbol for Breast Cancer Deaths by County 1970-1994.**

The layer symbol is the rectangle below the layer name in the table of contents.

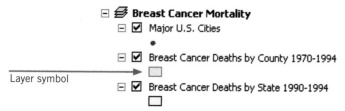

Layer symbol

2   In the resulting Symbol Selector window, click the Fill Color button in the Options frame.

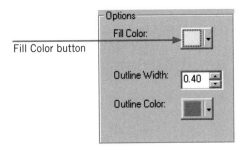

Fill Color button

3   In the color palette, click the Arctic White tile.

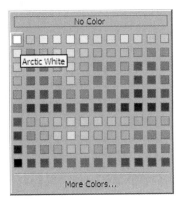

4   Click OK.

The layer's color will change to Arctic White on the map.

Change a layer's outline color

1   Click the layer symbol for Breast Cancer Deaths by County 1970-1994.

2   In the symbol selector, click the Outline Color button in the Options frame.

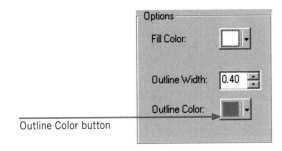

Outline Color button

3   In the color palette, click the Gray 20% tile.

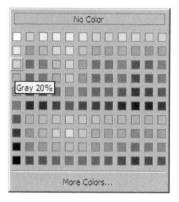

4   Click OK.

Change a layer's outline width

Because county and state boundaries share some lines, it is useful to display the U.S. states with a hollow fill and a dark, thick outline so you can see the county polygons above them.

1   Click the layer symbol for Breast Cancer Deaths by State 1990-1994.

2   In the Symbol Selector dialog box, click Hollow as the symbol.

3   In the Options frame of the Symbol Selector dialog box, click the box beside Outline Width.

4   Type **1.25** as the Outline Width and click OK.

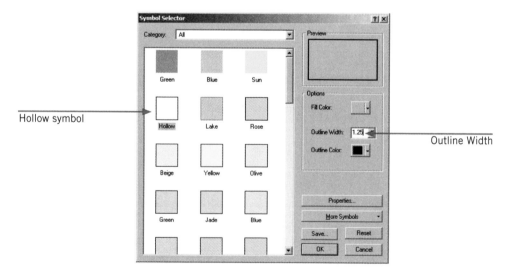

5   Move the **Breast Cancer Deaths by State 1990-1994** layer just above Breast Cancer Deaths by County 1970-1994 in the table of contents.

The resultant map is much easier to read. The layer names are self-descriptive, and it is easy to distinguish between the county and state outlines.

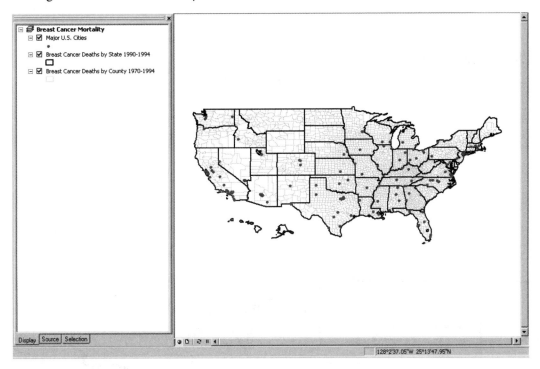

Zoom and pan health features on a map

Sometimes you will want to concentrate on a particular area of a map. Also, you will quickly learn that some geographic features are too small to see when viewing an entire map. If you enlarge a particular area, you can see the details more easily. Zooming and panning enlarges or reduces the display and shifts it to reveal different areas of the map. You will find zoom and pan buttons on the Tools toolbar.

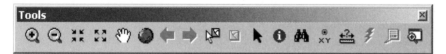

Zoom in

1   **Click the Zoom In button.**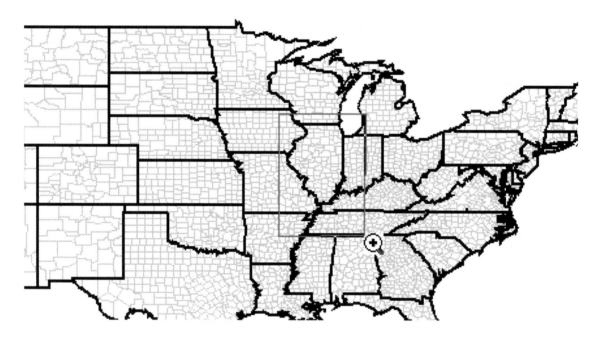

2   **Click and hold the mouse button on a point above and to the left of the state of Illinois.**

3   **Drag the mouse to draw a box around the state of Illinois. Release the mouse button.**

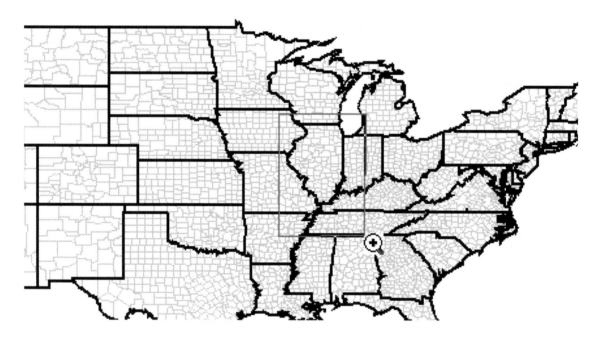

The resultant map is a zoomed area of the state of Illinois.

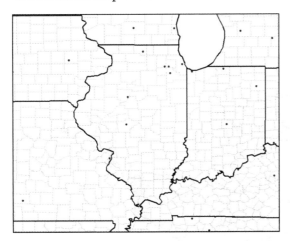

4   **Click the screen to zoom in, centered on the point that you clicked.**

Note: This is an alternative to dragging a rectangle for zooming in.

Pan

If you want to see a neighboring state without zooming out, use the Pan button.

1   **Click the Pan button.**

2   **Move the cursor anywhere onto the map view.**

3   **While holding the left mouse button, drag the mouse in any direction.**

4   **Release the mouse button.**

Panning shifts the current display to the left or right, up or down, without changing the current scale.

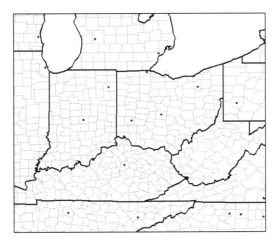

Zoom to full extent

If you want to zoom to the entire map, use the Full Extent button.

1   **Click the Full Extent button.**

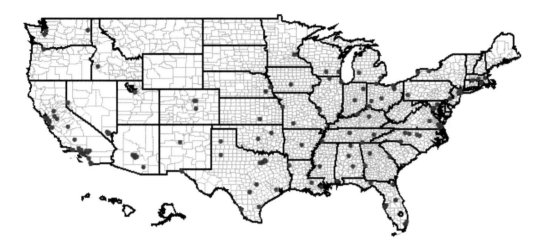

YOUR TURN

Practice using the other zoom functions such as a fixed zoom in and out, which zooms by a
fixed percent with each click. You can zoom back to the previous extent with the blue arrow on
the Tools toolbar.

Create spatial bookmarks

Spatial bookmarks save the current display, as zoomed in, with a name. You then can easily return to the saved area by accessing the bookmark. This is useful if you use GIS in presentations or to move quickly to a study area or region of interest.

1   Click the View menu and click Zoom Data, Full Extent.

2   Zoom to the state of Florida.

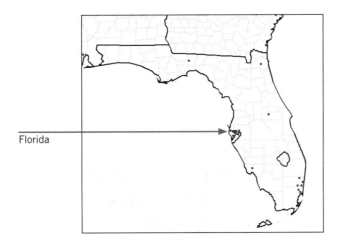

3   Click the Bookmarks menu, then click Create. Name the bookmark **Florida**.

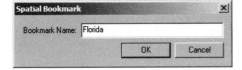

4   Click OK.

5   Click the View menu and click Zoom Data, Full Extent.

6   Click the Bookmarks menu, then select Florida.

ArcMap will zoom to the extent of the saved bookmark for Florida, which can be helpful if you frequently zoom to this extent.

YOUR TURN

Create spatial bookmarks for a few other states familiar to you. Then zoom to the full extent again.

Identify cancer mortality rates and deaths by state

With GIS you can interact with map layers to get information. The Identify tool is a commonly used point-and-click tool for browsing attribute data associated with the map feature. In this section you will use the Identify tool to learn about mortality rates and the number of breast cancer deaths per state and county.

Identify features

1   Turn off all layers except Breast Cancer Deaths by State 1990-1994.

2   From the Tools toolbar, click the Identify button.

3   Click inside the state of Texas.

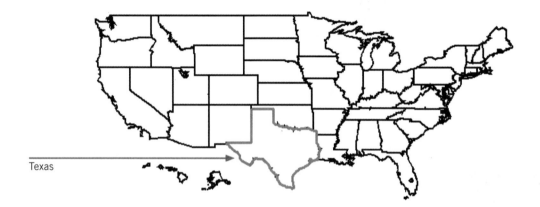

Texas

The state will temporarily flash and the results will appear in the resulting Identify dialog box.

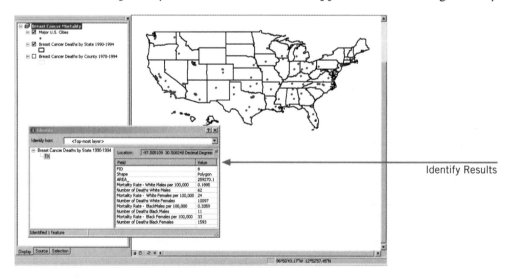

Identify Results

4   Click another state to see the cancer mortality rates and number of deaths.

5   Close the Identify dialog box.

If you have many layers turned on, you may have difficulty picking the appropriate feature to identify. For example you may pick a state instead of a county if both layers are on. To solve this problem you can restrict the identify selection to features in one layer only, ignoring features in the other layers.

1   Turn on the Breast Cancer Deaths by County 1970-1994 layer.

2   From the Tools toolbar, click the Identify button.

3   Click any state or county polygon feature.

4   Click the Identify from drop-down list in the Identify dialog box and click Breast Cancer Deaths by County 1970-1994.

This will restrict the identify selection to features in this layer only, ignoring features in the other layers.

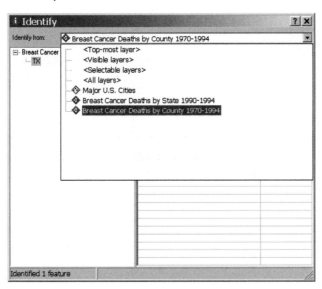

5   **Click any county polygon feature.**

The names of attributes use the following codes:

R=Mortality rate per 100,000 people, C=Number of deaths, WM=White Male,
WF=White Female, BM=Black Male, BF=Black Female, and 7094=1970-1994.

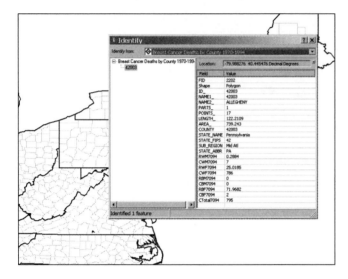

6   **Close the Identify dialog box.**

TURN

YOUR

> Practice using the Identify tool in a geographic area of interest to you. Restrict the layers to
> state, county, and major U.S. cities, and observe the data in each feature class. Are you able to
> observe any health-care phenomena?

Select map features

GIS links graphic features of a map layer with associated attribute records in a table. When you select features on a map, you can correlate them with the records in the table. In this way you can perform functions on a subset of features and records, such as generating statistics, making new layers, or doing analysis.

1   Turn off the Breast Cancer Deaths by County 1970-1994 layer.

2   Turn on the Major U.S. Cities layer.

3   From the Tools toolbar, click the Select Features button.

4   Click inside the Texas boundary.

The selected features highlight on the map.

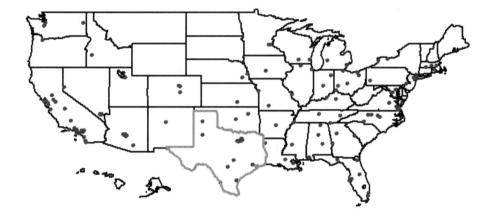

Select multiple features

1   To make multiple selections, hold the Shift key and click inside each of the states surrounding Texas.

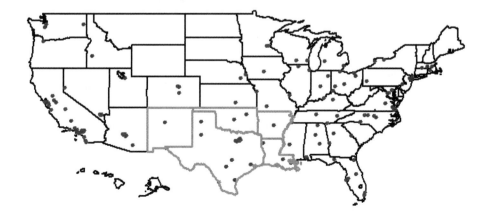

Zoom to selected features

1   Click the View menu and click Zoom Data, then Zoom to Selected Features.

ArcMap zooms to the features selected.

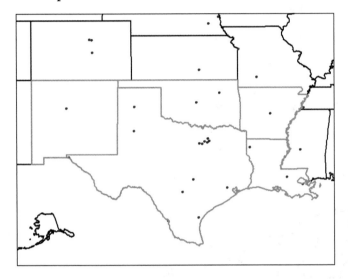

Clear selected features

1   Click the Selection menu and click Clear Selected Features.

2   Zoom to the full extent of the map.

YOUR TURN

Select features for five states in the northeast region of the United States, zoom to those selected features, and then clear the selection.

Change selection color

Sometimes a bright selection color is useful to better see selected map features.

1 **Click the Selection menu and click Options.**

2 **In the Selection Color frame, click the color button.**

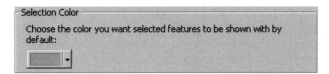

3 **Click Mars Red as the new selection color.**

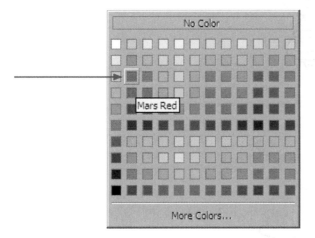

4 **Click OK.**

Change selectable layers

Similar to restricting layers to identify, you can restrict layers for selection. Making a layer selectable allows features to be selected with a variety of tools.

1 **Turn on all layers.**

2 **At the bottom of the table of contents, click the Selection tab.**

3 **Uncheck the boxes for Major U.S. Cities and Breast Cancer Deaths by State 1990-1994 to make them unselectable.**

4   Zoom to the northeast portion of the United States.

Only counties will be selectable now.

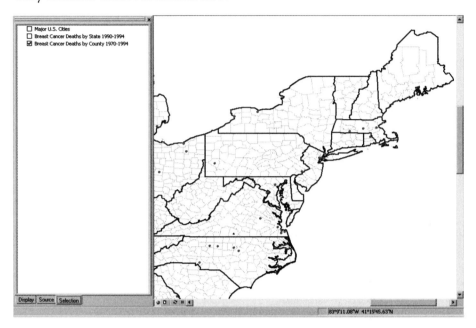

5   Click the Select Features button and **click a county.**

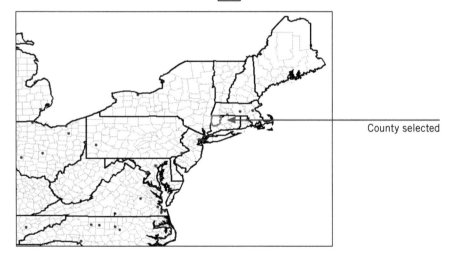

County selected

Notice that only a county is selected.

6   Clear the selected features.

YOUR TURN

Set the selectable layers to Major U.S. Cities and zoom to a state to select cities only. When you're done, be sure to clear the selected features and turn on all layers under the Selection tab, then change back to the Display tab in the table of contents.

Find map features

The connection between GIS features and their attributes provides several ways to locate features in the map. In cases where you know what you're looking for but don't know its location, you can use the Find tool.

1   **From the Tools toolbar, click the Find button.**

2   **Type Philadelphia in the Find box.**

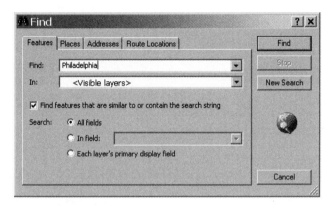

3   **Click Find.**

The results will appear in the Find dialog box. Note that ArcMap finds both the city and county of Philadelphia. These two records were located because the software searches all visible layers. You can restrict the Find tool to a specific layer by using the In drop-down list seen in step 2 above.

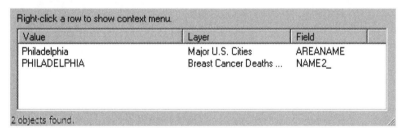

4   **Right-click the city name and click Zoom To.**

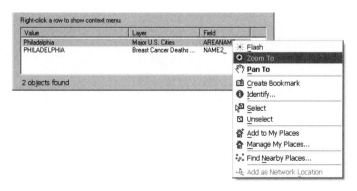

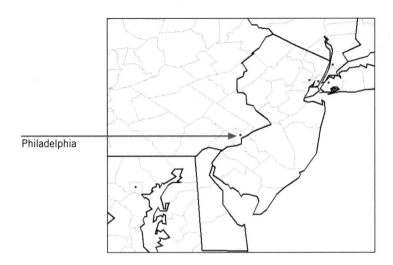

Philadelphia

5   **Close the Find dialog box and zoom to full extent.**

Use an attribute table to select counties with the highest number of breast cancer deaths

Every map layer has an associated feature attribute table that contains data associated with each feature in the layer. To explore the attributes of a layer on a map, open its attribute table. The attribute table provides information that you can use for queries. In this section you will use attribute tables to determine which U.S. counties have the highest number of breast cancer deaths.

Open an attribute table

1   In the table of contents, right-click the Breast Cancer Deaths by County 1970-1994 layer.

2   Click Open Attribute Table.

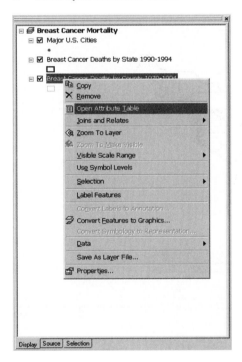

The table containing one record for each county feature opens. Every layer has such a table with one record per geographic feature.

3   Scroll down the table until you find Snyder County, Pennsylvania.

The order of records may be different on your computer than the one on the following page. Snyder County is number 2255 in the FID field. You will later learn how to select records by sorting fields.

4   Click the record selector (gray box) at the far left of the table to select that entire row.

5   Scroll to the right in the attribute table to see total deaths per county (CTotal7094).

Snyder County, Pennsylvania, is the county with the highest number of total breast cancer deaths from 1970 to 1994.

Record selector

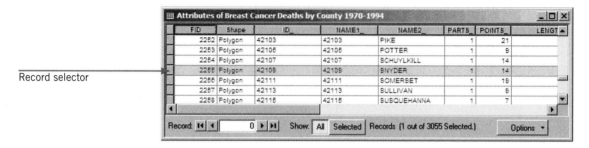

Show the connection between layers and tables

1   Resize the Attributes of Breast Cancer Deaths by County 1970-1994 table so that both the map and table on the screen can be viewed simultaneously.

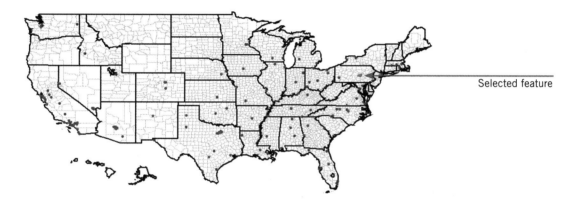

Selected feature

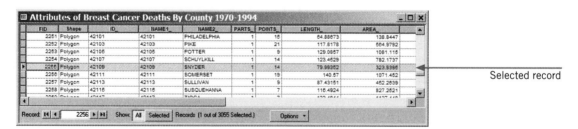

Selected record

2   Click various counties in the attribute table to highlight them in the map.

3   Click various counties on the map to highlight them in the feature attribute table.

YOUR TURN

Use the attribute table to find the county where you live. Select your county in the attribute table and see the county highlighted on the map.

Move a field

Next you will move and sort fields in the feature attribute table. In particular, you will sort fields in descending order by the total deaths in each county, and then select the highest number of deaths for the United States or for a selected state.

1　In the **Attributes of Breast Cancer Deaths by County 1970-1994** table, click the gray column heading (known as the field name) of the CTotal7094 field.

2　Click, hold, drag, and release the CTotal7094 field when it is to the right of the STATE_NAME field.

Column heading

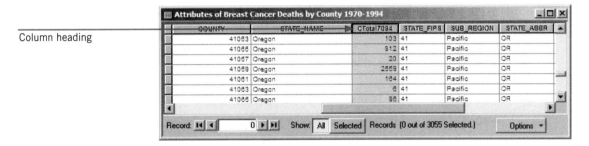

3　Move the STATE_NAME and CTotal7094 fields until they are to the immediate right of NAME2_.

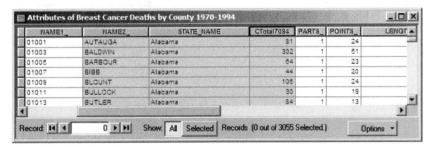

Sort a single field

1　In the **Attributes of Breast Cancer Deaths by County 1970-1994** table, right-click the CTotal7094 field name.

2　Click the Sort Descending button.

This will sort the table from the largest number to the smallest number of breast cancer deaths for each county.

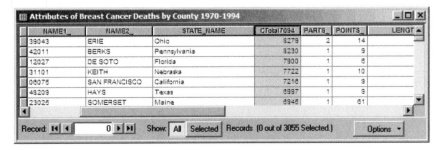

Select the top five counties

Now that you have prepared the attribute table to sort by the highest number of breast cancer deaths, you can select records to isolate top cancer counties on the map.

1   **In the Attributes of Breast Cancer Deaths by County 1970-1994 table, hold down the CTRL key and click row selectors for the first five records in descending order.**

Notice the corresponding features are highlighted on the map.

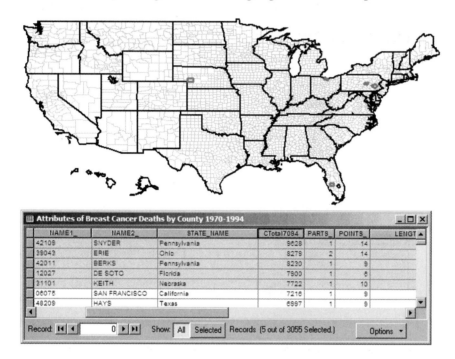

Show only selected records

1   **In the Attributes of Breast Cancer Deaths by County 1970-1994 table, click the Selected button.**

This will show only the records for the features selected in the map.

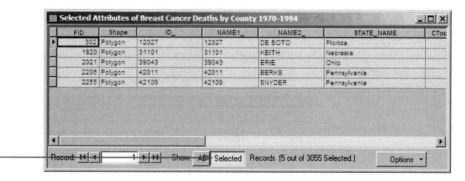

Selected Records

2   **Click the All button to show all records again.**

Clear selected records

1 In the Attributes of Breast Cancer Deaths by County 1970-1994 table, click the Options button at the bottom. [Options ▾]

2 Click Clear Selection.

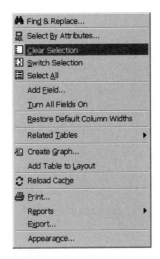

YOUR TURN

Sort the same attribute table by mortality rates for white females (field name RWF7094). Scroll through the table to see which counties have the highest mortality rate.

Sort multiple fields

Sorting by number of cancer deaths was useful for finding the counties with the highest number of breast cancer deaths and death rates across the United States, but what if you want to examine the number of deaths by state? To do this you would need to sort the records by two fields—state and number of deaths.

1 Hold down the CTRL key and click the STATE_NAME and CTotal7094 column headings to highlight both columns.

Be sure the CTotal7094 field is to the right of the STATE_NAME field.

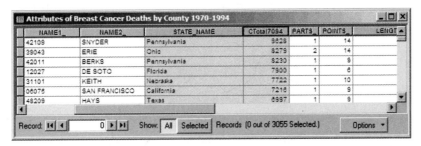

2   Right-click the STATE_NAME field and click Sort Ascending.

This will sort the field alphabetically by state name and then by breast cancer deaths.

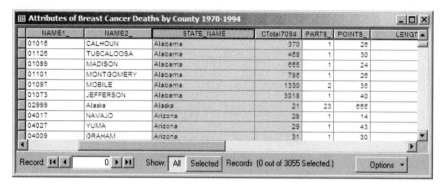

3   Scroll toward the bottom of the list until you find the records for Texas.

4   Scroll to the last of the records for Texas and select the five counties with the highest number of breast cancer deaths.

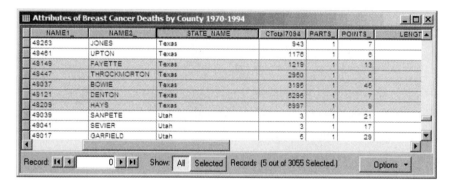

5   Click View, Zoom Data, Zoom to Selected Features.

The resultant map shows the locations of the top five counties with the highest number of breast cancer deaths in Texas.

6   Close the Attribute table.

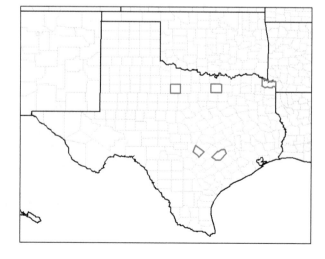

Create a new layer of a subset of features

Sometimes just a subset of features is needed in a map layer. For example, here you will select the most populated cities in Texas and make a new layer of just these cities.

Select the most populated cities

1   Open the Attributes of Major U.S. Cities table and click the POP2000 column heading.

2   Hold down the CTRL key and click the State (ST) field to highlight both fields. Be sure the Pop2000 field is to the right of the ST field.

3   Right-click the ST field and click Sort Ascending.

This will sort the field from the lowest populated city to the highest populated city. After sorting with multiple fields, you can easily select the most populated cities by state.

4   In the Attributes for Major U.S. Cities table, scroll toward the bottom of the table until you find the records for Texas.

5   Hold down the CTRL key and select the Texas cities whose population is over 500,000.

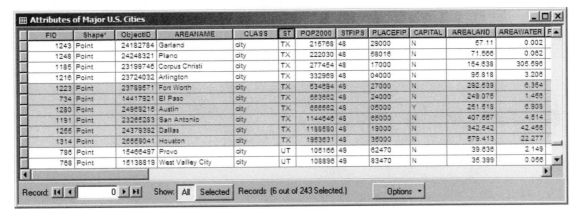

6   Close the Attributes of Major U.S. Cities table.

Create a layer from selected features

1   In the table of contents, right-click the Major U.S. Cities layer.

2   Click Selection, then select Create Layer from Selected Features.

A new layer of just the selected cities will be added to the table of contents.

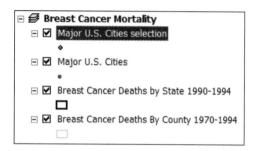

Create a new symbol for the new layer

The symbol should be changed to differentiate it from the other layer showing all Major U.S. Cities.

1   Right-click the Major U.S. Cities selection layer and click Properties.

2   Click the General tab and change the name of the layer to **Most Populated Texas Cities**.

3   Click the Symbology tab and the symbol button.

4   Change the symbol to a solid black circle. Set the size to 8 and click OK.

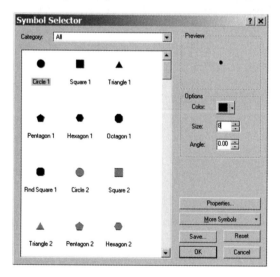

5   Click OK in the Properties dialog.

6   Turn the Major U.S. Cities layer off to show only the major cities in Texas, and zoom to the Most Populated Texas Cities layer.

7   **Zoom back to the extent of Texas.**

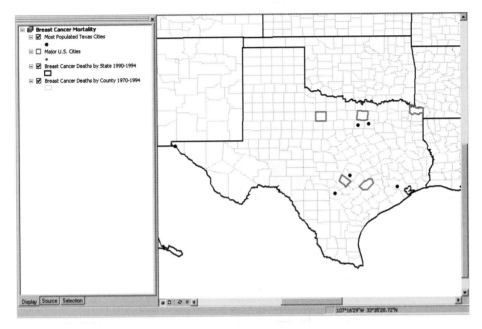

Label major cities in Texas

Sometimes labels are needed to inform the map reader about features they are seeing on a map, such as the major cities in Texas. Because GIS features are connected to attribute data in tables, you can easily label map features with any data found in the tables.

Set label properties and features

1   In the table of contents, right-click the Most Populated Texas Cities layer.

2   Click Properties.

3   Click the Labels tab.

4   Click the check box beside Label features in this layer.

5   Click the Label field drop-down arrow, and if necessary select AREANAME from the list of available fields.

6   Click Symbol, Properties, and the Mask tab.

7   Click Halo as the mask style.

8   Click Symbol and choose a bright yellow fill color.

9   Click OK three times.

10   Change the font to bold and the symbol size to 8.

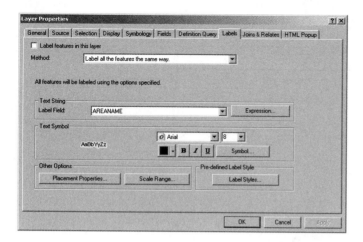

11 Click OK.

ArcMap labels the most populated Texas cities.

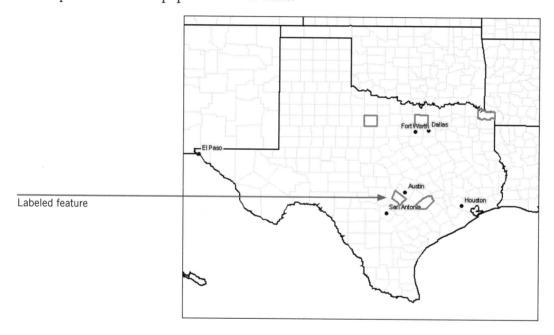

Remove labels

1   In the table of contents, right-click the Most Populated Texas Cities layer.

2   Click Label Features.

ArcMap turns the labels off.

3   Using the same procedure, click Label Features again to turn the labels back on.

Convert labels to annotations

Use labels to quickly generate maps showing text associated with a map feature. If you want to move individual labels, you need to convert labels to annotation text. Here you will convert the labels of Texas cities to annotations so that you can move them around the map.

1   In the table of contents, right-click the Most Populated Texas Cities layer.

2   Click Convert Labels to Annotation.

3   In the Store Annotation frame, click the radio button next to In the map.

Please note, if you had features selected you could choose Selected features in the Create Annotation frame to label only those selected.

4   Click Convert.

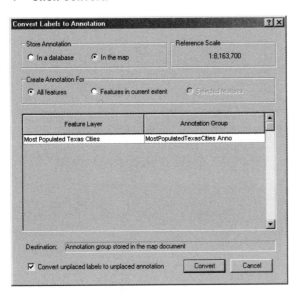

Move labels

1   Click View, Toolbars, and Draw.

2   On the Draw toolbar, click the Select Elements tool.

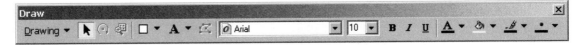

3   Click the labels for El Paso, Fort Worth, and Dallas, and using your own judgment, move the labels to better positions.

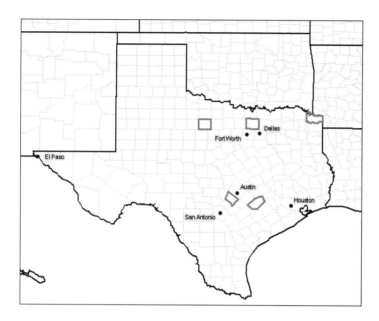

Save the project and exit ArcMap

1 **Click the File menu and click Save As.**

2 **Navigate to the \GistutorialHealth folder and save the map document as Tutorial2-1.mxd.**

This saves the current table and map information, including selected records and labels.

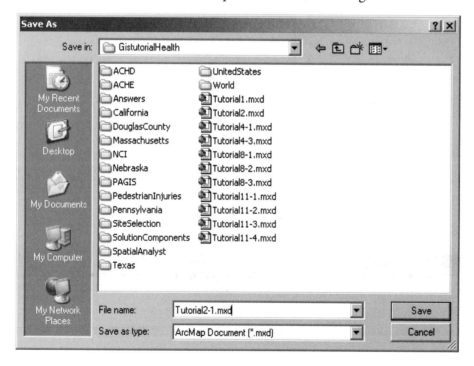

3 **Click the File menu and click Exit.**

Summary

You now have a good start on making ArcMap software work for you.

You have seen that a map document is composed of one or more map layers, added as needed and symbolized for the purpose at hand. You can symbolize map layers by changing colors, outlines, shapes, and so forth. You can also add labels or annotation to identify map features.

You can change the portion or extent of map layers you are viewing by zooming and panning. Spatial information is available at different scales. Some information, such as cancer mortality rates by state in the United States, can be gained when zoomed far out to the full extent of a map. Additional information, at a finer scale, is available by zooming to a state and viewing breast cancer mortality by county, with cities providing context. Zooming and panning are essential interactive tools for understanding both broad-brush and fine-detail information at different map scales. Sometimes you will find a close-up view of some features that you will want to revisit. In that case you can create a spatial bookmark for quickly jumping back to that view.

Each point, line, and polygon map layer is linked to a feature attribute table having as many attributes as are available and desired. You saw that each feature has its own data record, and if you select a map feature, ArcMap automatically selects its record. The opposite is true as well: if you select a table record, ArcMap selects its map feature. You can use the Identify, Select Features, Find, and Label tools to interact with features on your map.

Of course, you are working with map documents for a purpose—to find patterns and convey information about health, diseases, and related topics. The essential information comes from how the features are spatially arranged in the map layers and from the health data records that lie behind the features in the attribute tables. For example, you sorted breast cancer mortality rates for counties by state in the county attribute table, selected the top five counties in the state, and then viewed the spatial arrangement of the selected counties on the map with cities providing additional spatial context. These are unique and useful capabilities of GIS.

EXERCISES

Exercise assignment 2-1

Lung cancer mortality maps

Problem:

The National Cancer Institute (NCI) has a variety of Web sites to access cancer statistics and build interactive maps. Their Cancer Mortality Maps & Graph Web site, *www3.cancer.gov/atlasplus*, provides interactive maps, graphs, text, tables, and figures showing geographic patterns and time trends of cancer death rates for the time period 1950–1994 for more than 40 cancers. GIS maps and data can also be found on *gis.cancer.gov/nci /research.html* and *srab.cancer.gov/incidence/monograph.html*. These are excellent sites to build maps using pre-defined variables provided by the NCI. If you want to create more detailed or customized maps you need to use a desktop GIS application.

In this problem, you will use ArcMap to build a map showing lung cancer mortality for U.S. states and counties. You will use a GIS attribute table to determine the states and counties with the highest number of lung cancer deaths and then display them in a map.

Start with the following:

- **C:\GistutorialHealth\NCI\LungState5_9094.shp**—polygon shapefile of lung cancer statistics by state with attribute table data dictionary as follows:

Attribute	Definition
RWM90_94	mortality rate per 100,000, white males, 1990-1994
CWM90_94	number of lung cancer deaths, white males, 1990-1994
RWF90_94	mortality rate per 100,000, white females, 1990-1994
CWF90_94	number of lung cancer deaths, white females, 1990-1994
RBM90_94	mortality rate per 100,000, black males, 1990-1994
CBM90_94	number of lung cancer deaths, black males, 1990-1994
RBF90_94	mortality rate per 100,000, black females, 1990-1994
CBF90_94	number of lung cancer deaths, black females, 1990-1994
CTot90_94	number of lung cancer deaths, all, 1990-1994

Create a cancer mortality map for U.S. states

Create a new project called C:\GistutorialHealth\Answers\Assignment2\Assignment2-1.mxd with LungState5_9094 modified as a hollow fill, black outline, size 1.5.

Using the Attributes of LungState5_9094 table, select the following 10 Southeast, Mississippi Valley, and Gulf Coast states: Alabama, Arkansas, Florida, Georgia, Kentucky, Louisiana, Mississippi, Oklahoma, Tennessee, and Texas.

Show these in a bright red selection color. Label these selected states only with the state name or abbreviation and number of lung cancer deaths.

Create a Word document called C:\GistutorialHealth\Answers\Assignment2\Assignment2.doc. In it, create a table similar to the one below with statistics for the above selected states.

Hint:

Right-click each field in the Attributes of LungState5_9094 table to get needed statistics.

Variable	Total (Sum)	Maximum	Minimum	Mean
White Male				
Black Male				
White Female				
Black Female				

Save the project as C:\GistutorialHealth\Answers\Assignment2\Assignment2-1.mxd.

Exercise assignment 2-2

State lung cancer mortality maps

Problem:

Detailed maps for U.S. counties can also show some interesting patterns. The following observations are taken from the NCI, and you can use desktop GIS to explore these further.

- White males: Rates in the recent time period 1970-1994 were elevated across broad stretches of the Southeast, particularly along the Eastern Seaboard, across the Gulf Coast, and along the Mississippi Valley. Rates in the upper midwestern, Plains, and Rocky Mountain states were notably low, whereas rates in the northeastern and far western states approximated the national rate.
- Among white females, elevated rates during 1970-1994 tended to cluster along both the Atlantic and Pacific coasts, including most of Florida and California.
- Among black males and females, rates were high in scattered northeastern and midwestern areas, and low across much of the South.

Start with the following:

- **C:\GistutorialHealth\NCI\LungState5_9094.shp**—polygon shapefile of lung cancer statistics by state with attribute table data dictionary as follows:

Attribute	Definition
RWM90_94	mortality rate per 100,000, white males, 1990-1994
CWM90_94	number of lung cancer deaths, white males, 1990-1994
RWF90_94	mortality rate per 100,000, white females, 1990-1994
CWF90_94	number of lung cancer deaths, white females, 1990-1994
RBM90_94	mortality rate per 100,000, black males, 1990-1994
CBM90_94	number of lung cancer deaths, black males, 1990-1994
RBF90_94	mortality rate per 100,000, black females, 1990-1994
CBF90_94	number of lung cancer deaths, black females, 1990-1994
CTot90_94	number of lung cancer deaths, all, 1990-1994

- **C:\GistutorialHealth\NCI\LungCounty_7094.shp**—polygon shapefile of lung cancer statistics by county with attribute table data dictionary as follows:

Attribute	Definition
RWM70_94	mortality rate per 100,000, white males, 1970-1994
CWM70_94	number of lung cancer deaths, white males, 1970-1994
RWF70_94	mortality rate per 100,000, white females, 1970-1994
CWF70_94	number of lung cancer deaths, white females, 1970-1994
RBM70_94	mortality rate per 100,000, black males, 1970-1994
CBM70_94	number of lung cancer deaths, black males, 1970-1994
RBF70_94	mortality rate per 100,000, black females, 1970-1994
CBF70_94	number of lung cancer deaths, black females, 1970-1994

- **C:\GistutorialHealth\UnitedStates\MajorCities.shp**—point shapefile of U.S. cities with census demographics.

Create a detailed cancer mortality map for Illinois counties

Create a new project called C:\GistutorialHealth\Answers\Assignment2\Assignment2-2.mxd with the above layers for states, counties, and major cities. Zoom to Illinois and select the counties with black male lung cancer mortality rates over 100. Create a new layer of selected Illinois cities only. Label these cities with both the city name and population. Save your zoomed-in extent as a spatial bookmark so you can easily return to it.

Hints:

- Symbolize layers. Symbolize LungState5_9094 with a hollow fill, black outline, size 1.5. Symbolize LungCounty_7094 with a hollow fill, medium gray outline, and U.S. Cities with a black circle, size 6.
- Sort multiple fields (counties and total lung cancer deaths). Sort the LungCounty_7094 attribute table by both state name and mortality rate for black males.
  Hint: Move the RBM70_94 field to the right of the STATE_NAME field, highlight both fields by holding the CTRL key, then right-click the STATE_NAME field and choose Sort Ascending.
- Create a new layer from the selected Illinois cities. After selecting the cities, right-click the Cities layer and click Selection, Create Layer from Selected Features. Turn off the original cities and symbolize the selected cities with a dark blue circle, size 8. Convert the labels to annotation if you want to move or edit them.

Save the project as C:\GistutorialHealth\Answers\Assignment2\Assignment2-2.mxd.

What to turn in:

If you are working in a classroom setting with an instructor, you may be required to submit the exercises you created in tutorial 2. Below are the files you are required to turn in. Be sure to use a compression program such as PKZIP or WinZip to include all files as one ZIP document for review and grading. Include your name and assignment number in the ZIP document <YourNameAssignment2.zip>.

ArcMap projects

C:\GistutorialHealth\Answers\Assignment2\Assignment2-1.mxd
C:\GistutorialHealth\Answers\Assignment2\Assignment2-2.mxd

Word document

C:\GistutorialHealth\Assignments\Assignment2.doc

GIS Tutorial 3

Designing maps for a health study

Health-care scenario

Suppose that you have the ability to direct some state funds to help fund health-care costs for uninsured populations in Texas. Probably most uninsured are poor, so you want to investigate the correlation between uninsured populations and poverty indicators, including unemployment and minority status. You also want to locate the target populations on a map to see where funds would have to be concentrated.

Solution approach

Much of what needs to be done involves using cartographic (map design) principles to convey information about the underlying attributes of graphic features. So this section provides concepts and guidelines for that purpose.

The graphic elements available to symbolize maps include fill color and patterns for polygons; outline width, pattern, and color for lines—including outlines for polygons and point markers; and shape, size, and color for point markers. Maps cannot display continuous variation in numeric attributes because the human eye cannot readily interpret small changes in graphic elements. Instead, we must use large changes in graphic elements with approaches analogous to making bar charts for continuous variables in data tables.

An example is a choropleth map that uses solid fill color for polygons based on a relatively small number of intervals, covering the range of an attribute. The right-side boundaries of intervals are called break values and are included in their intervals, but left sides are not. For example, you will use 20 and less, 21–25, 26–30, and 31–35 for the percentage of uninsured persons per county in Texas, with break values 20, 25, 30, and 35. The interval 21–25 contains polygons with the percentage of uninsured greater than 21 and less than or equal to 25.

Except for the 0–20 interval, these are equal-width intervals wherein each covers a range of five percentage points. To make things easier to interpret, the break values were set to multiples of five. Taken as a whole, these intervals include, or span, the complete range of attributes stored for this variable. ArcMap has several other options for designing intervals. A helpful one for analysts uses quantiles that break up attribute values into equal-size groups. For example, for four intervals quantiles are the same as the more familiar quartiles, with each interval having 25 percent of the observations. Another useful option is to manually choose whatever break values you wish. Many phenomena have long-tail distributions to the right, with many low values and relatively few but far-ranging high values. (A long-tailed probability distribution is one that assigns relatively high probabilities to regions far from the mean or median.) In this case, a manual numeric scale using interval widths that double is often valuable; for example, 0–5, 5–15, 15–35, and 35–75, where the interval widths are 5, 10, 20, and 40.

The choice of colors for intervals is based on color value, which is the amount of black added to a color. A monochromatic color scale has a single color with light to medium to dark shades of the same color. Usually, the darker the color, the higher the interval of values; this makes it easy to interpret a map at a glance. Also, if you make a black-and-white copy of a map that has a monochromatic scale, the map will retain valid visual information through shades of gray. ArcMap software generates monochromatic and other color scales called color ramps. A design tip is to use monochromatic color ramps that have more light shades and fewer dark shades because the human eye is better at discriminating light shades.

The approach to symbolizing points depends more on variations in shape and size of point markers than color. A point is a mathematical object with no area, but to see a point on a map, we have to plot a point marker that does have area. Perhaps the most effective way to show variation in a numerical attribute of a point feature is to vary the size of a fixed-shape point marker, that is, use size-graduated point markers. For example, you might use five intervals and five circular point markers with increasing radii for increasing intervals. Often it is sufficient to use the same color for all sizes of point markers of an attribute, but you can also add a monochromatic color ramp to the fill color of point markers. Another design tip is to overexaggerate the differences in radii between successive point markers more than proportional increases in areas.

You will apply the above principles to studying the spatial pattern and correlation of uninsured and poor populations. The trick to plotting both on the same map is to use a county-based choropleth map for one variable and size-graduated point markers located at the centroids (center points) of counties for the other variable. ArcMap automatically creates the polygon centroids for the latter.

Often you will need to present your findings and write them up in reports. This calls for professional-quality, stand-alone maps suitable for these purposes, which is something beyond the interactive map views available in ArcMap software on a computer screen. As you may have guessed, ArcMap has the capacity to easily produce exactly what's needed using map layouts. Map layouts have all of the features necessary for using them outside of ArcMap: title, map, neatline, legend, scale bar, and so forth. A neatline places a border around a map, and the legend explains symbols and numeric scales used on a map. Scale is a graphic representation of distance, a straight line with a few distances marked off.

Begin a new map document

1   From the Windows taskbar, click Start, All Programs, ArcGIS, ArcMap.

2   Click the A new empty map radio button in the ArcMap dialog box.

3   Click OK.

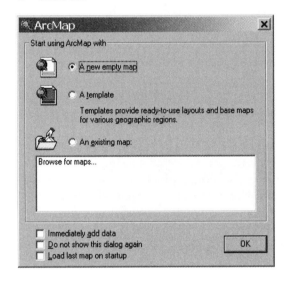

A new empty map is displayed. Next, you will add layers to the map and symbolize them.

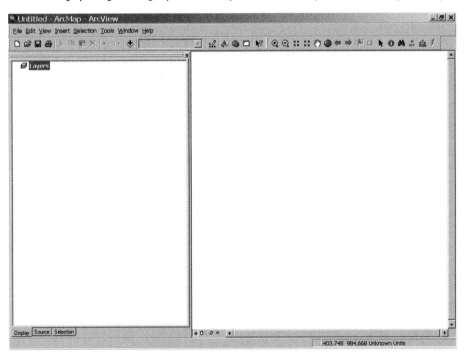

Create a choropleth map for the uninsured population in Texas

Your first task is to build a choropleth map for the percentage uninsured by county in Texas. As is the case with all symbolization in ArcMap, this process is highly automated so that you only have to make a few selections to render the entire map layer, rather than painting each graphic feature individually.

Add a layer and change its name

1 From the Standard toolbar, click the Add Data button.

2 Navigate to your **\GistutorialHealth** data folder and double-click the **\Texas** subfolder.

3 Click **Counties.shp** and click Add.

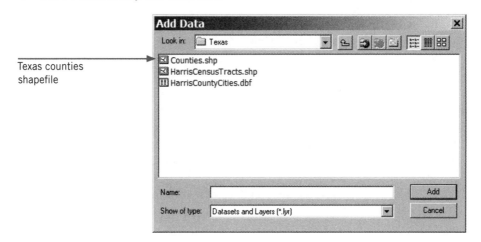

Texas counties shapefile

4 In the table of contents, right-click the Counties layer.

5 Click Properties.

6 Click the General tab.

7 Type **% of Population Uninsured** as the new layer name.

8 Click OK.

ArcMap picks an arbitrary fill color for the polygons. You will change the color later in the tutorial.

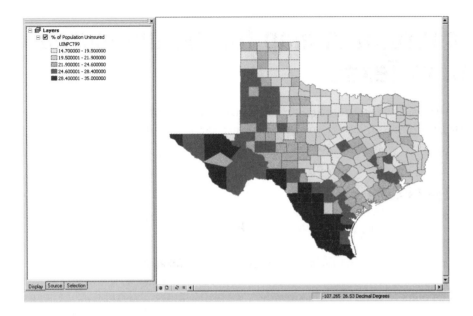

Select an attribute to display uninsured population

The Symbology tab in the Properties dialog box allows you to symbolize your data using unique colors for intervals covering the range of a numeric attribute among other options. There are several classification schemes to choose from. ArcMap Online Help describes all of the classification methods. Generally, it is best to use a monochromatic color scale, one color with increasingly darker shades progressing from small- to large-value intervals, or vice versa. Many prebuilt progressions of colors in ArcMap, called color ramps, are monochromatic. Here you will classify data for the percentage of uninsured people in Texas counties.

1   In the table of contents, right-click the % of Population Uninsured layer and click Properties.

2   Click the Symbology tab.

3   In the Show frame, click Quantities and click Graduated colors.

4   In the Fields frame, click the Value drop-down list and click UINPCT99.

Only numeric fields will appear in the Value drop-down list.

UNIPCT99 field

Graduated colors

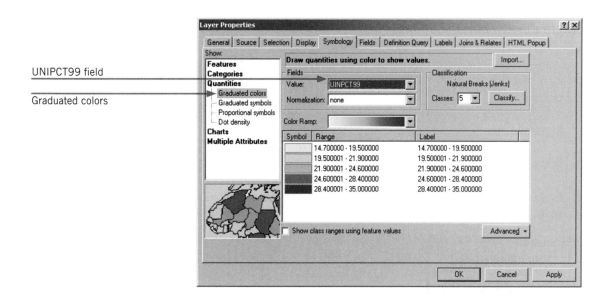

5   Click OK.

The result is five classifications of uninsured total population ranging from lowest to highest values with darker colors representing higher values. ArcMap picks an arbitrary color ramp and a particular method of creating intervals, called natural breaks, for the polygons. You will learn how to change the colors and classification methods later.

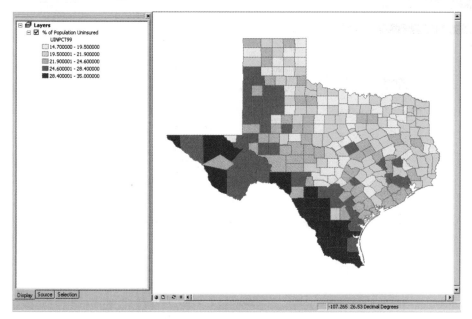

Create custom classifications

One of the powerful features of desktop GIS is the ability to create your own custom classifications and to choose or modify color ramps. You will create your own custom legend here for the percentage of population that is uninsured.

1   **Right-click the % Population Uninsured layer and click Properties.**

2   **In the Layer Properties dialog box, click the Symbology tab.**

3   **In the Classification frame, click the Classes drop-down arrow and change the number of classes to 4.**

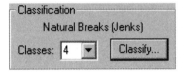

4   **In the Classification frame, click the Classify button.**

The Classification dialog box shows the current classifications, statistics, and a histogram of the data with current classification break values listed.

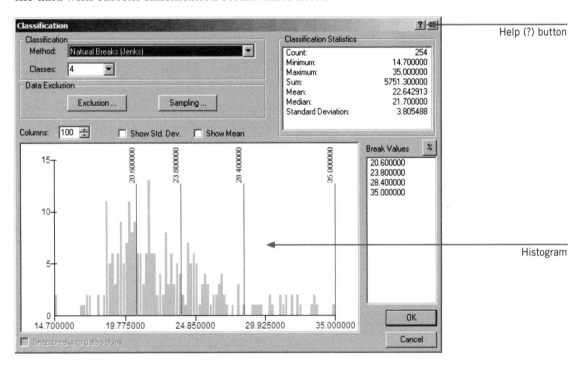

5   **Click the Help (?) button in the upper right corner of the dialog box (shown above).**

6   **Click any area of the dialog box to learn more about that section.**

Manually change classification values for percentage uninsured

The next task is to break up the range of uninsured population into intervals, such as you would do if you were making a bar chart for these data.

1   In the Classification frame, click the Method drop-down list, then click Manual.

2   In the Break Values panel, click the first value, 20.600000, to highlight it.

Notice that the blue line in the graph corresponding to that value turns red.

3   Type **20** and press the Enter key to move to the next break value.

4   Continue the same pattern to create the following break values: **25**, **30**, and **35**.

5   Click OK.

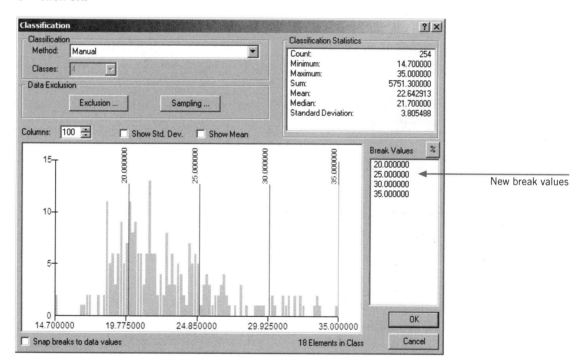

Change labels

1   Within the Symbology tab of the Layer Properties dialog box, click the Label button.

2   **Click Format Labels.**

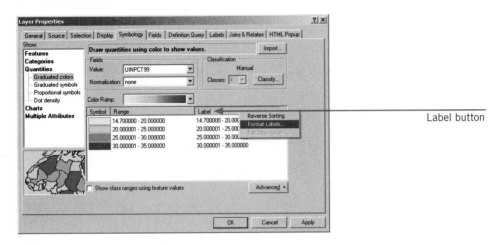

Label button

3   **Click Percentage in the Category panel.**

4   **Click the Numeric Options button.**

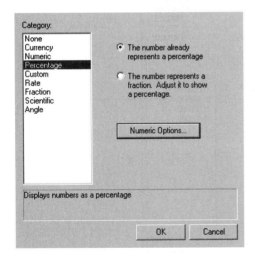

5   **Set the Number of decimal places to 0 and click OK. Click OK again.**

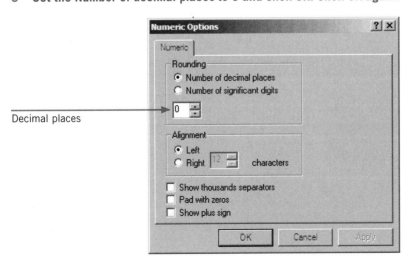

Decimal places

6   Change the first label value to under 20%.

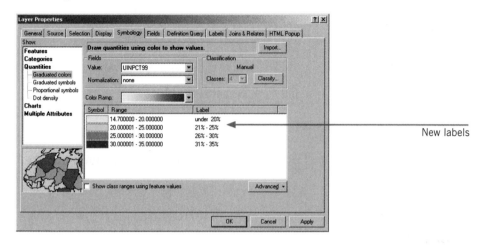

New labels

7   Click OK.

The changes to the layer's legend, using fixed intervals of width 5, have made the map easier for lay audiences to interpret.

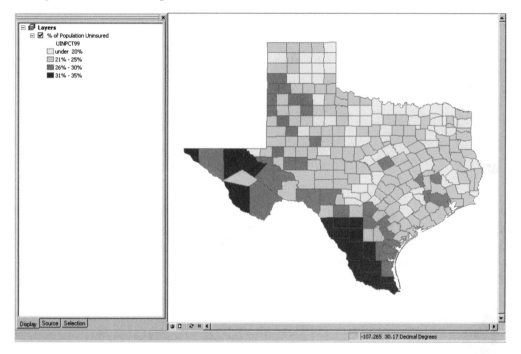

Build a custom color ramp

Generally, it is best to have more classes with lighter colors and a few with darker colors because the human eye can differentiate lighter colors more easily than darker colors. Next you will build a custom color ramp with lighter colors.

1   Right-click the % Population Uninsured layer and click Properties.

2   In the Layer Properties dialog box, click the Symbology tab.

3   Click the Color Ramp drop-down arrow, scroll to the top, and click the fourth color ramp from the top (shades of blue).

4   Right-click the Color Ramp and click Properties.

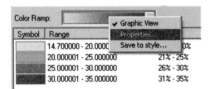

5   Click the color box to the right of Color 1 and click Arctic White.

6   Click the color box to the right of Color 2 and click Dark Navy.

7   Click OK twice.

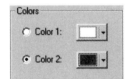

The % Population Uninsured map now has a new, custom color ramp, ranging from white to dark blue. You can also double-click each color box in the Symbology tab of a map layer's properties dialog box to change the classification colors individually.

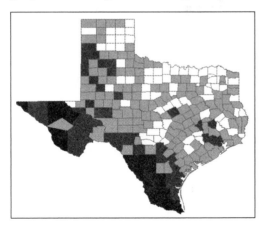

Save the Texas health-study map

8   Click File then Save As.

9   Save the map as **\GistutorialHealth\TexasHealthStudy.mxd.**

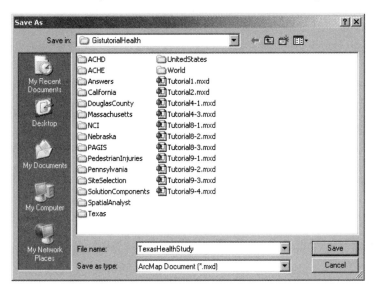

Create a point map for percentage of unemployed in Texas

Here you will add unemployment data as points to your uninsured choropleth map so you can look for a correlation between the unemployment rate and the number of people without health insurance. To show variation in unemployment, you will break up that variable's range into intervals, similar to those for the insured, but this time you will use the point-marker size instead of a color ramp to differentiate the intervals. The larger the size, the larger the interval's value.

Symbolize unemployment data as graduated points

1   If it is not already opened, open the map document that you created with the choropleth map, **\GistutorialHealth\TexasHealthStudy.mxd**.

2   Again add the data layer **\GistutorialHealth\Texas\Counties.shp** to your current project.

3   Double-click Counties to open the Layer Properties.

4   Click the General tab and change the name of the layer to **% of Population Unemployed**.

5   Click the Symbology tab.

6   In the Show panel, click Quantities, Graduated symbols.

7   In the Fields frame, change the Value to PCTUNEMP.

8   Change the Template symbol to a red circle, the Symbol Size to a range of 2–24, and the Background fill and the Outline to no color.

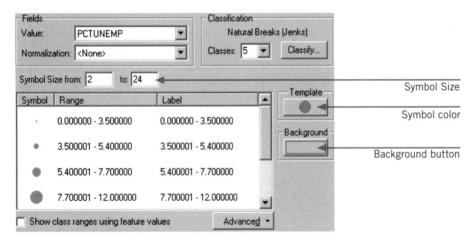

9   Click OK.

Modify point classifications

The default classifications for the points need to be modified so an even comparison to the uninsured can be made.

1   **Double-click % of Population Unemployed to open the Layer Properties.**

2   **Click the Symbology tab and click the Classify button.**

3   **From the Method drop-down list, click Equal Interval.**

The resultant intervals break values are not whole numbers. To make the numeric scale easier to interpret, you will manually adjust the break values to even intervals of a width of 4.

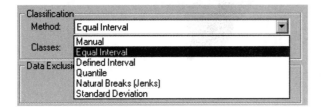

4   **Change the break values to 4, 8, 12, 16, and 20 and click OK.**

5   **Change the labels to under 4%, 4% - 8%, 8% - 12%, 12% - 16%, and 16% - 20.9%.**

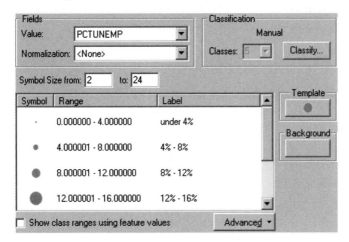

6   **Click OK.**

The resultant map on the next page shows the counties layer twice, once as a choropleth map with graduated colors and once as a point map with graduated points. You can see the direct correlation between the unemployed and uninsured populations: there is a tendency for both to increase together.

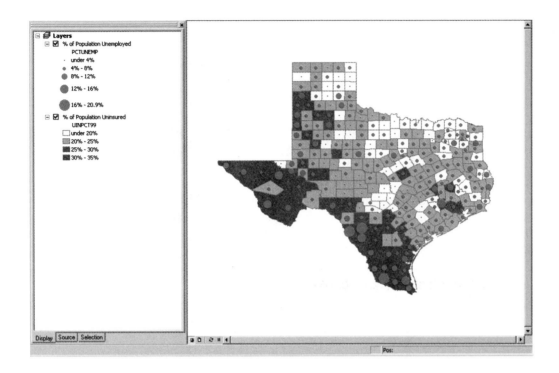

Make a scatter plot comparing uninsured and unemployed populations

Scatter plots display pairs of attributes and may reveal a relationship between the values plotted. Here you will create a scatter plot showing the positive correlation between uninsured and unemployed.

1   Click the Tools menu, click Graphs then Create.

2   In the Graph type drop-down list of the Create Graph Wizard, click the Scatter Plot icon.

3   In the Y field drop-down list, scroll down and click UNIPCT99.

4   In the X field (optional) drop-down list, scroll down and click PCTUNEMP.

5   Uncheck Add to Legend.

6   Click Next.

7   In the Title box, type **Relationship of Uninsured and Unemployed Populations**.

8   Uncheck the Graph legend option.

9   In the Axis properties Left Title panel, type **Percentage Uninsured**.

10   In the Bottom Title panel, type **Percentage Unemployed**.

11   Click Finish.

The result is a scatter plot that helps to summarize and support the results of the correlation between unemployed and uninsured. Right-clicking anywhere on the graph opens a context menu that allows you to make revisions to your graph by clicking Advanced properties or Properties. For example, you can add the graph to the layout of your current map or export it to a variety of graphic formats. You can also use Microsoft Excel with Counties.dbf in the Texas folder to calculate the correlation coefficient of these two variables, which is quite strong at 0.66. If you do manipulate this file with Excel, do not save any of your changes to Counties.dbf, as doing so could corrupt the link between the spatial and attribute data.

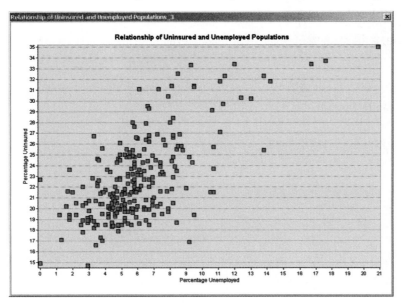

Save the changes to your Texas health-study map

1   Click File, Save As.

2   Save the project as **\GistutorialHealth\TexasHealthStudy2.mxd**.

Work with layer files

ArcMap has features that allow you to save and reuse your symbology, including classification schemes, colors of choropleth maps, and graduated point markers. To do this, you can save a layer's symbology to a layer (.lyr) file. These layer files allow you to use the same layer symbology across several maps.

Create a layer file

1   In the **TexasHealthStudy map**, right-click % of Population Unemployed.

2   Click Save As Layer File.

3   Navigate to the **\GistutorialHealth\Texas** folder.

4   Type **Unemployed.lyr** as the layer file name to save.

5   Click Save.

YOUR TURN

Save the % of Population Uninsured layer to a file called Uninsured.lyr, also located in the Texas folder.

Create a group layer and add saved layers

You can also group several layers into a "group layer" whose layers can be turned on and off with one click of the mouse.

1   **Click File then New. In the New dialog box, click the My Templates tab, then click Blank Document and OK.**

2   **Right-click Layers in the table of contents.**

3   **Click New Group Layer.**

4   **Right-click the resulting New Group Layer and click Properties.**

5   **Click the General tab.**

6   **Type Texas Unemployment/Uninsured Comparison as the group layer name.**

7   **Click the Group tab.**

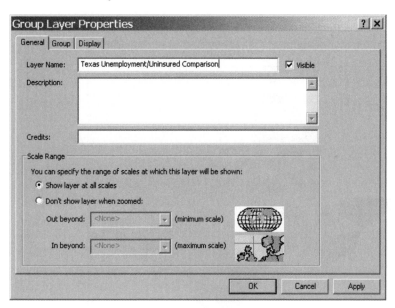

8   **Click the Add button.**

9   **Navigate to \GistutorialHealth\Texas.**

10 While holding the Shift key, click **Unemployed.lyr** and **Uninsured.lyr**, Add, and OK.

The resultant map document displays the already-symbolized Texas polygon and point features comparing unemployed and uninsured in a layer group.

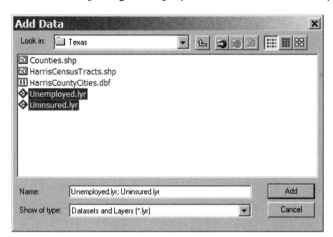

11 Collapse the tree structure of the existing layers in the table of contents by clicking the leftmost boxes that have minus signs (-) for % of Population Uninsured and % of Population Unemployed.

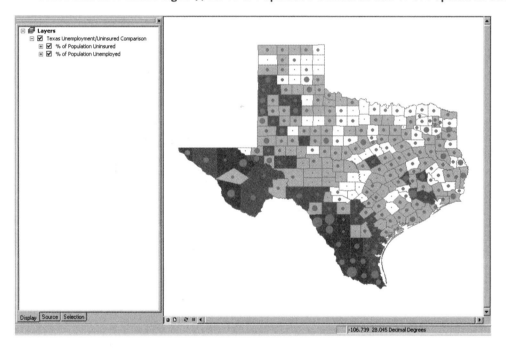

You can reverse this process by clicking again the boxes that now have plus signs (+) indicating that they can be expanded.

YOUR TURN

Turn the existing group layer off and create a new group layer called Texas Uninsured/Hispanic Population Comparison. Add the Uninsured.lyr file that you saved. Add the Counties.shp layer again, this time showing the number of Hispanic people in Texas (field HISPANIC) as graduated points. Save this layer called C:\GistutorialHealth\Texas\HispanicPopulation.lyr. You will use this layer file in an upcoming task.

Save the new Texas health-study map

1   Click File, Save.

2   Save the project as \GistutorialHealth\TexasHealthStudy3.mxd.

Print layouts for a health-care study

Often, you will want to produce a paper copy or file copy of a map for distribution or use in a report or presentation. For such a use, you will want to have a stand-alone map with a title, map, legend, and possibly other components. ArcMap has a Layout View for this purpose and several prebuilt templates for producing layouts.

Choose a prebuilt layout template

1   Click File, New to begin an ArcMap document.

Be sure to click File, New—otherwise the dialog box for layout templates will not appear.

2   Click the General tab.

3   Click **LetterLandscape.mxt** as the map layout template and click **OK**.

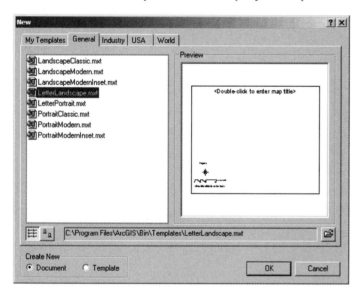

A premade map layout appears. Next, you simply need to add layers to the template.

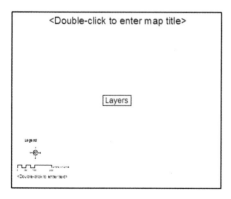

Add layers to the map layout

1 Click the Add Data button.

2 Navigate to **\GistutorialHealth\Texas** and add the layers **Uninsured.lyr** and **Unemployment.lyr**.

3 Double-click the title and change it to **Texas Uninsured and Unemployment Comparison**.

You may need to change the font size to fit the text on the map.

4 Delete the North Arrow and Map Scale, which are not necessary for this map.

5 Double-click the word Legend. In the Legend Properties dialog box, click the Legend tab, and delete the word Legend.

6 Click the Items tab and add % of Population Unemployed and % of Population Uninsured to the legend items.

7 Click OK.

8 Use the Select Elements tool ▶ from the Draw toolbar to move the legend to the lower left corner of the map layout and resize the legend.

9 Click the Fixed Zoom Out ⬚ button on the Tools toolbar.

10 Double-click the <Double-click to enter text> box that's in the lower left portion of the template, and type **Data obtained from U.S. Census Bureau, 2000**, click OK, then move the text to the right edge of the layout.

11 Save the project as **\GistutorialHealth\TexasHealthStudyLayout.mxd**.

The resultant layout is suitable for many uses.

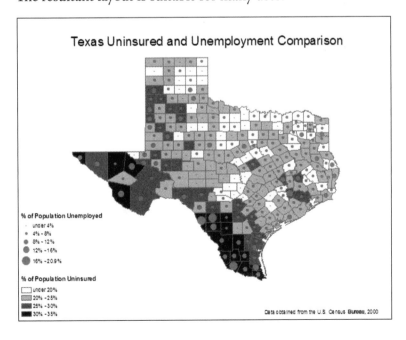

Create custom map layouts for multiple maps

To facilitate comparisons, it is often effective to place two or more maps on the same layout. Choose the same classification break values when comparing similar maps. For example, if you want to compare uninsured minority populations, such as African-Americans and Hispanics, use the same break values for both populations.

To create multiple maps, you need to create multiple data frames. A data frame is a fundamental element in a map. When you create a map, it contains a default data frame listed in the table of contents where you add layer files.

Build a custom layout grid

1   From the Standard toolbar, click the New Map File button.

2   Click View, Layout View.

3   Right-click the border of the Layout, click Page and Print Setup.

4   In the Page frame, change the standard size to Legal and click the Landscape radio button. Click OK.

5   Click the horizontal ruler at the 0.5-, 5.5-, 6.0-, 11.0-, and 13.5-inch marks.

6   Click the vertical ruler at the 1.5- and 7.0-inch marks.

7   Click and drag the layer frame so that its upper left corner snaps to the intersection of 0.5-inch horizontal guide and the 7.0-inch vertical guide.

8   Click and drag the lower right grab handle of the data frame to snap it at the 5.5-inch horizontal guide and the 1.5-inch vertical guide.

The layout should look like the following.

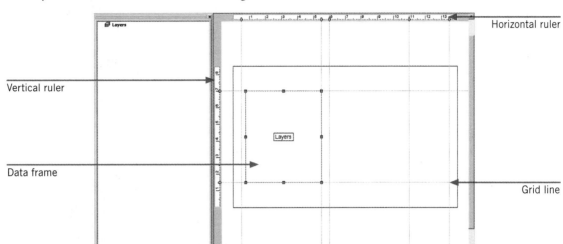

Horizontal ruler

Vertical ruler

Data frame

Grid line

Add layers and create multiple data frames

In one data frame you will add Uninsured and Hispanic populations. In a second data frame you will add Uninsured and Black populations.

1   Click the Add Data button, browse to **\GistutorialHealth\Texas**, and add **Uninsured.lyr** and **HispanicPopulation.lyr**.

2   Click Insert, Data Frame, and drag/modify the new data frame to fit in the guides beside the original frame.

3   Click the Add Data button, browse to **\GistutorialHealth\Texas**, and add **Uninsured.lyr**.

4   Click the Add Data button and add the shapefile **\GistutorialHealth\Texas\Counties.shp**.

The resulting layer in the new data frame is a single color and needs to be classified. When you have more than one data frame in a map, you need to be aware of which data frame is active. Many of the ArcMap tools and commands work only on the active data frame. The active data frame is the frame that is highlighted with the blue boxes on the layout page. Its name also appears in bold in the table of contents. You can click another data frame to make it active or right-click the data frame in the table of contents and click Activate.

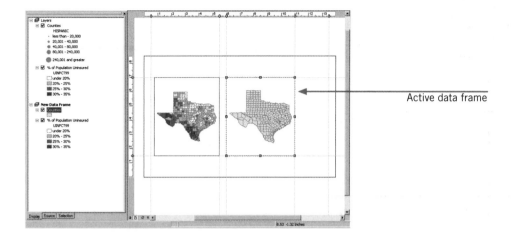

Active data frame

Classify data

1   In the table of contents, double-click the Counties layer and choose the Symbology tab.

2   Click the Import button.

3   From the Import Symbology dialog box, click the browse button to load an existing layer file.

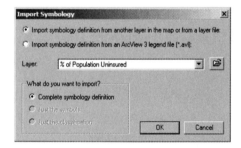

4   Click the **HispanicPopulation.lyr** file, Add, and OK.

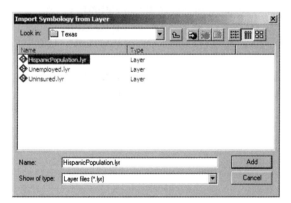

5   Click Counties as the layer in the Import Symbology dialog box, and OK.

6 Click the Value Field drop-down arrow, Black, and OK.

7 Click OK in the Layer Properties dialog box.

This will show the Black Population of Texas with the same classification as the Hispanic Population. Both maps will show the same uninsured map layer.

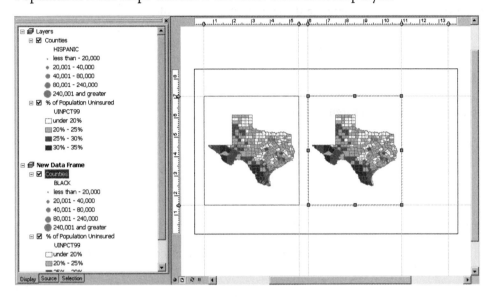

Rename data frames

Similar to layers, you can rename a data frame and change other properties.

1 In the table of contents, right-click the original data frame (currently named Layers) and click Properties.

2 Click the General tab and type **Hispanic Population Compared to Uninsured** in the Name box, then click OK.

3 Rename the other data frame **Black Population Compared to Uninsured**.

Add map titles and text

You need to add an overall title and titles for both data frames. The overall title should be in larger type.

1 Click Insert, Title.

2 Type **Texas Minority Population Compared to Uninsured, 2000** as the title.

3 Change the symbol font to bold, size 28 and move the title to the appropriate location on the layout.

4 Click Insert, Title.

5 Type **Hispanic Population and Uninsured.**

6 Change the symbol font size to 18 and place the title just above the corresponding data frame in the layout.

YOUR TURN

Create a title for the Black Population and Uninsured data frame and add text for the data source (U.S. Census Bureau, 2000).

Add a legend

If you want precise control over the legend elements created by ArcMap, you can convert a legend to graphics and edit individual legend elements. The legend created by ArcMap is dynamic and automatically will reflect any changes that you make to symbolization. However, a legend converted to graphics is static and will not reflect subsequent changes to symbolization. Here you will convert your legend to graphics so you can delete the field names in the legend. If deleting field names isn't necessary, you can use the Legend Properties dialog box to modify your legends.

1 **Click Insert, Legend.**

2 **Click Next four times and then Finish.**

3 **Move the legend to the lower right corner of the page and resize it to fit the available space.**

4 **Right-click the legend and click Convert to Graphics.**

5 **Right-click the legend again and click Ungroup.**

This allows you to edit individual parts of the legend.

6 **Double-click the title of the population legend and change it to Total Number of People.**

7 **Delete other unnecessary text such as the word Legend and field names such as UINPCT99.**

8 **Save the map document as \GistutorialHealth\TexasHealthStudyLayoutComparison.mxd.**

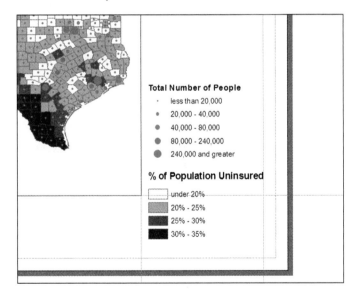

Unify map scales

You need to set the map scales for both data frames so they are exactly the same. Otherwise, one map may be slightly larger than the other, thus biasing the map reader to that map.

1   **Click in the Hispanic Population data frame to make it active.**

2   **Click in the scale box beside the add data button.**

3   **Type the scale 1:13,000,000, then press Enter.**

Scale box

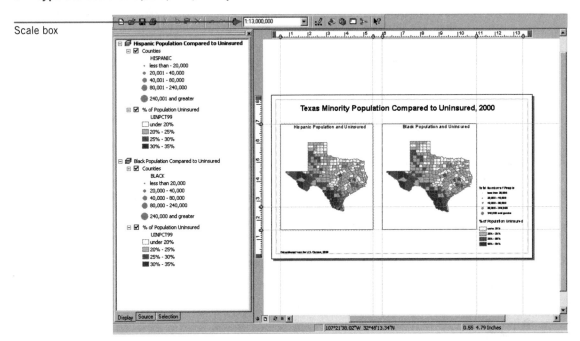

YOUR TURN

Set the scale for the Black Population data frame also to 1:13,000,000, so that it matches the first data frame scale.

Congratulations! You just created a sophisticated map layout that compares two maps. Other map elements that might be interesting to add to the map include a neatline (border around the map), bar charts or other charts, or photographs.

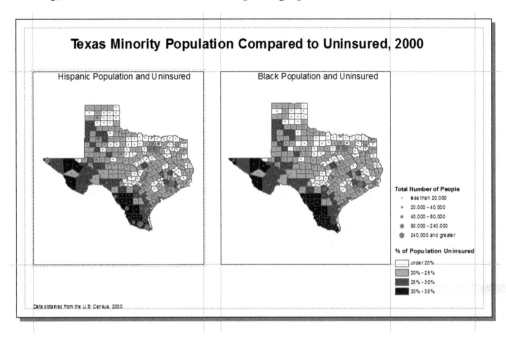

Save the Texas health-study map

1 Click File, Save As.

2 Save the project as **GistutorialHealth\TexasHealthStudyLayoutComparison.mxd.**

Export maps

Often you will need to share your maps with others or use maps with other software for presentation or publication. You can export ArcMap maps to many image formats, or map elements can simply be copied and pasted into other applications such as a Microsoft Word document, Microsoft PowerPoint presentation, or Web page.

Export a map to an image file

1   From the map layout, click File, then Export Map.

2   Click the Save as type drop-down arrow and click TIFF.

3   Navigate to **\GistutorialHealth\Texas** and save the file as **TexasHealthStudyLayoutComparison.tif.**

Other common image types include raster formats, JPEG, bitmap, PNG, and GIF. Other export types include Adobe PDF (Portable Document Format) software and vector formats AI (Adobe Illustrator), SVG (Scalable Vector Graphics), and EPS (Encapsulated Postscript).

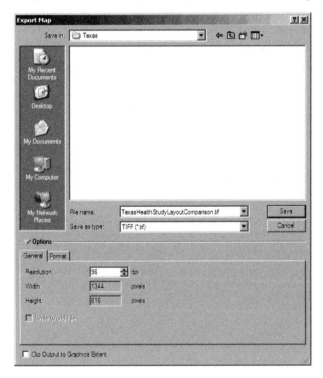

TURN

Export the map layout to a PDF file.

Copy and paste map images

You will often use maps in PowerPoint presentations or in Word documents, and it may be better to copy the map components individually. This allows you to edit parts of the map in PowerPoint or Word. Be aware that some map symbols may not appear properly if your presentation is shown on a computer without ArcMap (or ESRI symbols).

1   While in the map layout, click in one of the data frames.

You will see blue grip boxes around the data frame.

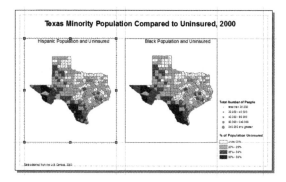

2   Press the CTRL and C keys at the same time.

3   Launch another application such as PowerPoint or Word.

4   Click Edit, Paste.

The map element will be pasted into the application and you can edit it there.

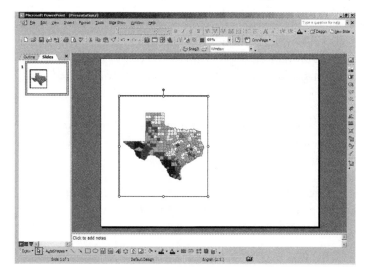

YOUR TURN

Copy and paste map elements from the rest of the map layout to your Word or PowerPoint application.

Summary

The mapping exercise in this tutorial revealed some interesting and perhaps useful patterns of uninsured populations in Texas. First, you saw as expected a high correlation between being uninsured and being poor. The maps that you made, however, further showed that much of the poverty and unemployed population is along the border of Texas and Mexico. The location of Hispanic and African-American minority populations—often among the poor—seems less a factor in explaining locations of uninsured populations. Further research is needed to better understand this preliminary result.

In this tutorial you learned to symbolize maps using numeric attributes of points and polygons. Unless you are working in the transportation area, you will rarely use lines, such as streets and rivers, for more than spatial context. So lines generally have background colors in analytic mapping. You learned about numeric scales for designing intervals to cover the range of attributes. Equal-width intervals, quantiles, and increasing-width intervals are commonly used in mapping. Visual rendering of numeric intervals uses monochromatic color ramps for polygons and size-graduated point markers for points.

Presentations and reports are the primary outlets for the health-care maps that you design in ArcMap. You will want to communicate your findings to policy and decision makers, and the best vehicle for that purpose is a map layout. You can very easily use ArcMap to generate professional map layouts that make a map a stand-alone product. Included in a layout is the map or maps, a title, distance scale, legend for interpreting symbols, and so forth. You simply export map layouts as image files and insert them into Word documents or PowerPoint presentations.

Besides teaching you how to build map layouts, this tutorial has also advanced your map design skills with sophisticated maps that allow for comparisons of two variables—in this case, the percentage of uninsured per county versus the percentage unemployed or percentage minority population. You learned how to create choropleth and graduated point-marker maps, which can be viewed together in the same map composition. Moreover, you found that map layouts with two such map compositions side-by-side, allow for comparison of three variables at the same time. You found a correlation of uninsured populations and poverty indicators, as expected, but the map provided further information on where and how intensely clustered the health-insurance problem is.

ArcMap is a very flexible software package, allowing much custom mapping. You created custom break points for choropleth and graduated point-marker maps, making the maps easy to interpret because of the uniform scales used.

Now you are in a good position to create effective interactive maps in ArcGIS in order to explore and research important spatial patterns. Plus you have the skills to convert finished maps into map products for others to understand and use.

Exercise assignment 3-1

Map comparing uninsured populations in California counties

Problem:

State of California officials suspect that counties with the highest number of uninsured populations correspond with other census variables such as households with single moms or African-American and Hispanic populations. Your task is to make GIS maps comparing this data.

Start with the following:

- **C:\GistutorialHealth\California\Counties.shp**—polygon shapefile of California counties.

  Attributes of Counties Fields:
  BLACK—Total Black/African-American population
  HISPANIC—Total Hispanic/Latino population
  UINTOT—Total number of uninsured population
  UINTOT18—Total number of uninsured under age 18
  FHH_CHILD—Total number of households with a woman and children but no husband

Create a choropleth and pin map

Create a new project called C:\GistutorialHealth\Answers\Assignment3\Assignment3-1.mxd showing three maps in a layout comparing the uninsured population to census variables for African-American, Hispanic, and female head of households with children (single moms). Think carefully about your color, point, pattern, or classification schemes so each variable is clearly understood. Be sure to rename the data frame and layers.

Export the layout as a PDF file called C:\GistutorialHealth\Answers\Assignment3\Assignment3-1.pdf.

Hint:

To show the population as points, choose graduated symbols as the quantities and choose a hollow background without an outline. ArcMap will use the centroid of the county polygon as the point.

EXERCISES

Exercise assignment 3-2

Map showing detailed Texas county demographics

Problem:

In addition to displaying and analyzing GIS data at a state level, analysts can also create demographic maps for a smaller geographic area such as a county, city, or neighborhood. For example, basic population and housing data is available for U.S. census tracts and block groups, which are subdivisions of counties. An interesting study would be to see the current population and housing status of Harris County, Texas, where Houston is located. In 2005, refugees from Hurricane Katrina moved to this city and some plan to permanently relocate there. This will likely cause some economic and health-related stresses to that area, and GIS maps can help public officials prepare for possible problems.

Start with the following:

- **C:\GistutorialHealth\Texas\HarrisCensusTracts.shp**—polygon shapefile of Harris County census tracts.

  Attributes of Harris Census Tracts fields:
  POPO4_SQMI—2004 population density per square mile
  VACANT—Number of vacant housing units
  RENTER_OCC—Number of renter occupied housing units

- **C:\GistutorialHealth\Texas\HarrisCountyCities.shp**—point shapefile of cities in Harris County.

Create choropleth maps

Create a new project called C:\GistutorialHealth\Answers\Assignment3\Assignment3-2.mxd comparing the three variables from the above census tracts shapefile in a map layout. Add the Harris County Cities for reference. Think carefully about your color, point, pattern, or classification schemes so each variable is clearly understood. Be sure to rename the data frame and layers.

Export the layout as a JPEG file called C:\GistutorialHealth\Answers\Assignment3\Assignment3-2.jpg.

Question:
In a Word document called C:\GistutorialHealth\Answers\Assignment3\Assignment3.doc, answer the following questions:
1. What observations can be made by comparing the above attributes?
2. What other census data would be good to compare and why?

What to turn in:

If you are working in a classroom setting with an instructor, you may be required to submit the exercises you created in tutorial 3. Below are the files you are required to turn in. Be sure to use a compression program such as PKZIP or WinZip to include all files as one ZIP document for review and grading. Include your name and assignment number in the ZIP document <YourNameAssignment3.zip>.

ArcMap projects
C:\GistutorialHealth\Answers\Assignment3\Assignment3-1.mxd
C:\GistutorialHealth\Answers\Assignment3\Assignment3-2.mxd

Word document
C:\GistutorialHealth\Answers\Assignment3\Assignment3.doc

Exported maps
C:\GistutorialHealth\Answers\Assignment3\Assignment3-1.pdf
C:\GistutorialHealth\Answers\Assignment3\Assignment3-2.jpg

OBJECTIVES

Project maps for health-data analysis at different geographic scales
Prepare incidence and prevalence maps
Import and project map layers for a local analysis

GIS Tutorial 4

Projecting and using spatial data

Health-care scenarios

This tutorial has three health scenarios, or applications, allowing us to discuss and demonstrate map projections appropriate for health studies at the world, continental, and local levels. In addition, we include assorted GIS topics that arise naturally at different geographic scales.

In the first scenario, a public health official working for an international health organization wants to study a snapshot of AIDS data for the entire world. For example, the enormity of the AIDS problem is well-known for sub-Saharan Africa. AIDS has created 13.2 million orphans in that part of the world and the Joint United Nations Program on HIV/AIDS estimates that by 2010 there will be more than 42 million orphans there—the number of children living in the United States east of the Mississippi River. The public health official would like to have a map that clearly identifies other heavily impacted parts of the world.

The second scenario is a brief revisit to the U.S. map showing male lung cancer mortality by county, seen as figure 1.1 in tutorial 1. We use this map solely to demonstrate various map projections for the continental United States.

The third scenario involves the municipal and neighborhood levels. The client is a task force of universities, schools, and health-care organizations working on reducing childhood obesity in Pittsburgh, Pennsylvania. Members of the task force want a map of parks and other areas used for outdoor activities around public schools. The map could be used for designing school physical fitness programs.

Solution approach

The smaller the map scale—or the more of the world included on a map—the more distortions appear in projected flat maps. Some combination of area, shape, direction, or distance is always distorted for maps of the world, hemispheres, continents, and large countries. As map scale increases to the state or province level and municipal level, distortions decrease because planes become good approximations of the earth's surface in very small areas. Nevertheless, mapmakers need to choose which projection to use for maps at all scales. For example, a good projection for a map of the world is the Robinson projection; a good one for the continental United States and displaying disease incidence is the Albers equal area conic projection; and good projections for substate areas of the United States are the state plane and universal transverse Mercator (UTM) projections—although there are many other good projections and considerations in making choices (see ArcMap Help for more information about choosing projections).

One important side issue regarding small-scale maps is the display of count data by area. An example is disease incidence, which counts disease cases by area and within a time interval. Disease incidence is valuable for gauging the size of a health problem and corresponding needs for funding, supplies, or facilities. As you know from tutorials 1 and 3, choropleth maps are commonly used for such data.

Perceived meaning in choropleth maps comes from two signals: color value (or the darkness of a color's shade) carries the primary information, but polygon size is a secondary and possibly false signal. The viewer's perception may be overly influenced by large polygons with high color value, while small polygons with high color value may be just as important, or even more important. For example, if a large and a small polygon have roughly the same large number of cases, they both will have the same high color value, but the smaller polygon will have more cases per square mile. If contagion is a factor in contracting the disease, then the smaller polygon may be more important.

In addition to this inherent nature of choropleth maps, small-scale maps potentially can have large and systematic errors in polygon areas.

The remedy is to limit your use of small-scale choropleth maps and instead use size-graduated point markers located at polygon centroids to symbolize variables such as disease incidence. Then point-marker size is the only variable, with no confusion or distortion. An exception is made for medium-scale maps (i.e., the size of the continental United States), for which good equal-area projections are available that remove projection-induced errors in area. Figure 1 in tutorial 1 uses such a projection. The choropleth map shows county boundaries, which are numerous and relatively small so that area does not carry much information and color value sends clear signals. In this case, graduated point markers are too numerous to see and interpret, unless the viewer zooms into a section of the country.

Disease prevalence of a communicable disease, represented as cases per 10,000 people, provides information about the extent of communicable disease diffusion throughout a population. With this measure, a small country with high prevalence will show up prominently, whereas, a large country with low prevalence but high raw count of cases will show up less prominently—the opposite of a map with just raw counts. Again, graduated point markers located at polygon centroids are preferable to choropleth maps.

Next, we discuss how ArcMap and ArcCatalog handle map projections—a major topic of this tutorial. A map document can have one or more data frames in its table of contents. The GIS user can switch between data frames in data view and a map in layout view to display separate maps for any or all data frames of the map document. Each data frame has its own collection of map layers and a projection.

A data frame can have map layers, each with its own projection, as long as each map layer has a spatial reference—data recording its projections and coordinate system. Then ArcMap has the information to reproject map layers to the data frame's projection on-the-fly for display. If the GIS analyst wishes to change a data frame's projection, he or she may do so and ArcMap will reproject all the data frame's map layers to the new common projection whenever the map document is opened.

Many spatial data formats, including those used in personal geodatabases and shapefiles, have spatial references (i.e., projections or coordinate systems). For example, a shapefile can have a projection file, and a personal geodatabase can have a geodatabase feature class in a table that stores spatial references. If you have a map layer that does not have a spatial reference, but you know its projection and coordinate system, you can use ArcCatalog to add the spatial reference to the map layer.

Small-scale maps of the world and country generally use relatively few and readily available basemap layers—for example, political boundaries such as countries, states or provinces, and counties or other political subdivisions. In contrast, large-scale maps, such as for a city or neighborhood, often require detailed map layers from several local sources. Acquired map layers can be in any of several data formats—all of which ArcCatalog or ArcMap can import, transform, or use directly. Some commonly encountered vector data formats, which you will use in this tutorial, include the following:

- *ArcInfo coverage*—An older data format for earlier GIS products that places each map layer in its own folder containing several files. Many organizations still keep their map layers in this format.
- *.e00 interchange file*—An even older data format that places an ArcInfo coverage into a single file, instead of a folder of files, for ease of transfer.
- *Shapefile*—A widely used data format with three or more files per map layer, each with the same file name but different extensions (e.g., .shp, .dbf, .shx).
- *Geodatabase*—The latest spatial data format commonly used, with all map data stored in relational database format. The personal geodatabase is built into ArcGIS and uses the Microsoft Access database engine. ArcSDE software, another ESRI product, uses enterprise-level database packages with ArcGIS. Databases from Oracle or Informix are used for geodatabases.
- *CAD*—Drawings made from computer-aided design (CAD) software applications. Many architectural or engineering firms create and use CAD files to create GIS base layers. ArcMap can add CAD files in one of two formats: native AutoCAD (DWG), Drawing Exchange Files (DXF), or Microstation (DGN).
- *Event tables*—A table for point features that includes attributes for x,y coordinates. Some organizations include coordinates with point data, making it easy to map the data with any GIS package. Global Positioning System (GPS) data is a source of event data—for example, showing the location of a truck as a series of points over time. ArcMap can directly display event table data as points.

With this background in hand, it's time to work on the tutorial.

Explore map projections for world AIDS study

In this section you will create a map comparing estimates of the cumulative number of AIDS cases in countries across the world.

Open an existing map

You will begin by opening the map document Tutorial4-1.mxd, which has three data frames, each with the same two map layers already symbolized. When you open the map document, all three data frames are unprojected, with geographic, latitude–longitude coordinates. You will set the first data frame to the Mercator projection, the second to the cylindrical equal-area projection, and the last to the Robinson projection.

1   From the Windows taskbar, click Start, All Programs, ArcGIS, ArcMap.

2   In the resulting ArcMap window, click the An existing map radio button and click OK.

3   Browse to the drive and folder on which the **\GistutorialHealth** folder is installed (e.g., **C:\GistutorialHealth**).

4   Click the **Tutorial4-1.mxd** document icon and click Open.

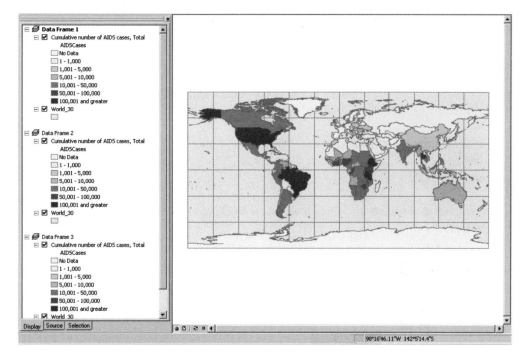

Change Data Frame 1's projection to Mercator

1   In the table of contents, right-click Data Frame 1 and click Activate.

This action activates the map layers in Data Frame 1 for use in the map. Only one data frame can be active at a time. You will activate the other two data frames in turn. Notice that the cursor in the graphic below is close to the (0,0) coordinate in the geographic coordinate system as seen in the coordinates field at the bottom of the map document window.

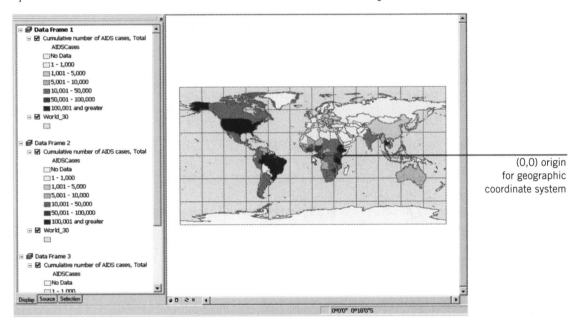

(0,0) origin for geographic coordinate system

2   Move your cursor around the map from the origin to the west, east, north, and south to see the range of values for the geographic coordinate system.

3   In the table of contents, right-click Data Frame 1 and click Properties.

4   Click the Coordinate System tab.

5   In the Select a coordinate system box, click the plus sign (+) next to the Predefined folder to expand its contents.

Expanded view of the Predefined folder

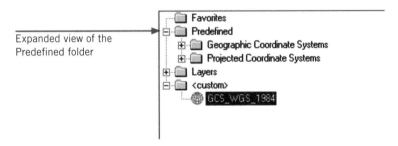

6   Inside the Predefined folder, expand the Projected Coordinate Systems folder, and then expand
the World folder.

Expanded view of
the World folder

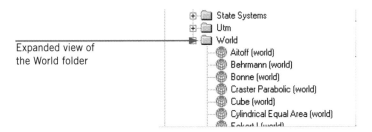

7   Scroll down, click Mercator, and click OK.

8   In the table of contents, click the Data Frame 1 title, wait a second or two, click it again, and type
Mercator Projection to change the name of the data frame.

9   Click View, Zoom Data, Full Extent.

The resultant map shows world AIDS cases using a Mercator projection. Notice how large
Greenland and Antarctica are! These are enormous distortions.

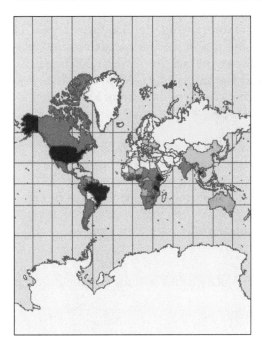

YOUR TURN

Repeat the above steps applying the cylindrical equal-area projection to Data Frame 2 and
the Robinson projection to Data Frame 3. Recall that the Mercator is a conformal projection,
preserving direction; the cylindrical equal-area projection preserves area; and the Robinson
projection is a hybrid that minimizes the misrepresentation of shape, area, distance, and
direction by allowing small amounts of distortion in each of these spatial properties. When
finished, save your map document as GistutorialHealth\Tutorial4-1.mxd.

Symbolize area maps using size-graduated point markers

Frequency data, such as the number of AIDS cases, is better shown by using graduated point markers for polygon centroids rather than choropleth maps. In this section you will show the number of world AIDS cases using graduated point markers and the Robinson projection.

Start a new map document

1   Click File, New, My Templates, Blank Document, and OK to begin a new map document.

2   Right-click the Layers data frame in the table of contents and click Properties.

3   Click the Coordinate System tab and click Predefined, Projected Coordinate Systems, World, Robinson (world), and OK.

Each map layer you will add in the next step is a shapefile that includes a projection file with the .prj extension. These files store the projection and coordinate information of a shapefile.

The coordinates of the shapefiles you will load are geographic (latitude and longitude). When you add the shapefiles, ArcMap reads the information in the projection file to determine their projection and coordinates, then spatially adjusts the data to match the projection defined for the data frame, which you just defined as Robinson. The ability of ArcMap to read a projection file and automatically adjust spatial data according to the data frame's projection is referred to as "on-the-fly projection."

On-the-fly projection is extremely useful when you are working with data layers stored in different projections and you need those layers to correctly overlay each other in the map. Keep in mind that on-the-fly projection is a temporary adjustment to the data that occurs only within the map document—it does not permanently alter the coordinates of the layers.

4   Click the Add Data button and add the **\GistutorialHealth\World\AIDSCases.shp** and **World_30.shp** layers.

The World_30 layer contains a graticule made up of lines of constant latitude and longitude at 30° intervals.

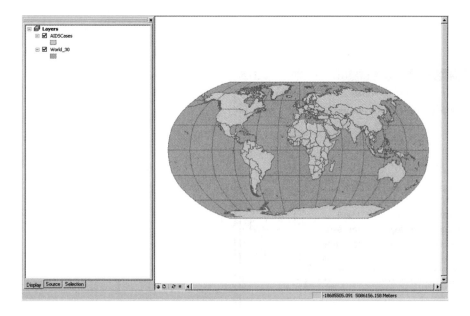

Symbolize layers

1　Right-click AIDSCases in the table of contents, click Properties, and click the Symbology tab.

2　In the Show panel, click Quantities and Graduated symbols.

3　In the Fields frame, click the Value drop-down arrow, and click AIDSCases.

4　Use the Template button to change the symbol type to Circle 2 with a red fill color.

5　On the Symbology tab, set the symbol size range to 2–12.

6　Use the Background button to set the background to white.

7　Use the Classify button to define 7 classes with manual break values of **0**, **1000**, **5000**, **10000**, **50000**, **100000**, and **900000**.

8　In the Layer Properties dialog box, double-click the smallest red point-marker symbol for the 0 class, and change the point marker to Circle 1 with no fill color.

This step makes the point marker for the 0 class invisible.

9   In the Layer Properties dialog box, click the Label heading above the label area, click Format Labels, change the number of decimal places to 0, and click OK. Click OK again.

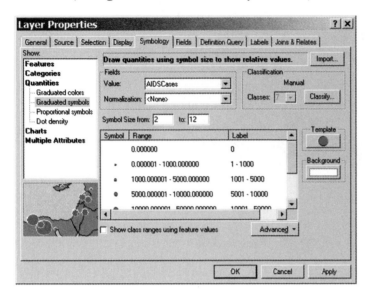

10   Symbolize the World_30 layer with a light blue fill color.

11   In the table of contents, click each layer's name and then, in a second or two, click it again to activate the text cursor, and type in labels as seen below (**Cumulative AIDS Cases, 30 Degree Graticule**).

Dark fill color in country polygons, seen at the beginning of this tutorial, made for false perceptions. For example, the United States' AIDS problem was overblown and Eastern Europe's was understated. This map, however, clearly shows the volume of AIDS cases by countries of the world, with heavy concentrations in sub-Sahara Africa and a surprising number in Eastern Europe.

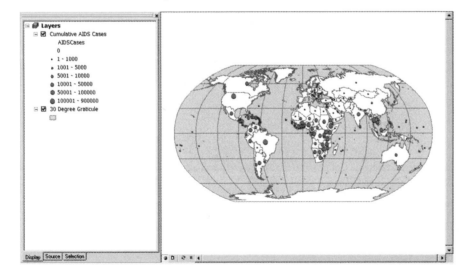

12   Save the map document as **\GistutorialHealth\Tutorial4-2.mxd.**

Create a prevalence map using point markers

Prevalence maps help to illustrate the progression of an infectious disease. Here you will map AIDS prevalence (rate per 10,000 people) using graduated point symbols and the Robinson projection. First, you will calculate the prevalence by creating a new field for the incidence rate.

1   In the **Tutorial4-2.mxd** map document, right-click Cumulative AIDS Cases and click Copy.

2   Click Edit, Paste, and turn off (uncheck) the second copy of that layer in the table of contents.

3   Right-click the first copy of Cumulative AIDS Cases and click Open Attribute Table.

4   In the Attributes of Cumulative Aids Cases, click Options, Add Field.

5   Name the new field **AIDSRate**, set its Type as Double, then click OK.

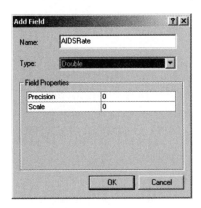

6   Scroll to the right end of the attribute table, right-click the AIDSRate field name, click Field Calculator, and click Yes.

7   In the Field Calculator, scroll down the Fields list, double-click AIDSCases, click the multiplication (*) button, type **10000**, click the division (/) button, double-click POP_CNTRY, and click OK.

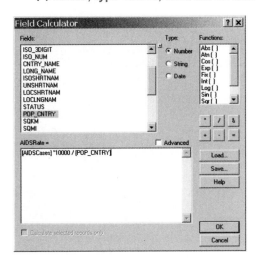

The resultant attribute table shows the prevalence of AIDS per 10,000 people.

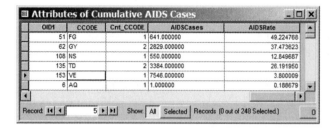

Attributes of Cumulative AIDS Cases

OID1	CCODE	Cnt_CCODE	AIDSCases	AIDSRate
51	FG	1	641.000000	49.224768
62	GY	2	2829.000000	37.473623
108	NS	1	550.000000	12.849687
135	TD	2	3384.000000	26.191950
153	VE	1	7546.000000	3.800009
6	AQ	1	1.000000	0.188679

Record: 5   Show: All Selected   Records (0 out of 248 Selected.)   0

TURN YOUR

Symbolize the top layer to yield AIDS prevalence per 10,000 people as seen below. Compare the two portrayals of AIDS: incidence and prevalence. There are some notable differences. Save the map document as Tutorial4-2.mxd.

This map shows the alarming scope of AIDS in sub-Saharan countries and the Caribbean, deemphasizing most of the rest of the world, compared to the previous map on incidence.

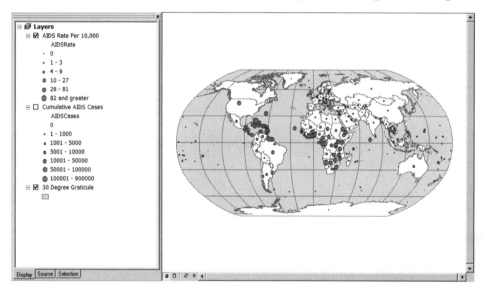

8 **Save the map document.**

Explore map projections for a U.S. lung cancer study

Here you will explore projections for the 48 states of the continental United States. You already know how to change the projection of a data frame, so you will just open a finished map document in layout view and observe differences in the projections. The spatial reference used for the geographic coordinates data frame is in the Data Frame Properties, Coordinate System tab under Predefined, Geographic, North American Datum 1983. For the two U.S. contiguous projections, see Predefined, Projected Coordinate Systems, Continental, North America.

YOUR TURN

> Open Tutorial4-3.mxd, a map document with four data frames in layout view for the contiguous 48 states. Study differences in the projections. The geographic coordinates flatten the map in the north–south direction. Both the equal-area and equidistant projections are comparable in appearance and good choices for use. We used the equal-area conic projection for figure 1.1 of tutorial 1 with the same data. The Robinson projection, while very attractive for viewing the entire world, has undesirable distortions for viewing the United States by itself.
>
> To add the table of contents to the map document (if it is not visible and you wish to use it), click Window and Table of Contents. To access the Tools toolbar, click View, Toolbars, and Tools. To see the data view, click View and Data View.

Geographic Coordinates

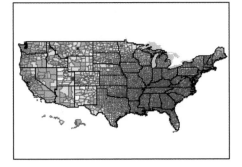

USA Contiguous
Albers Equal Area Conic

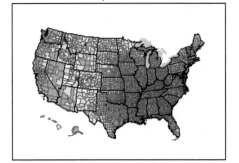

World Robinson

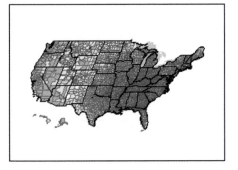

USA Contiguous
Equidistant Conic

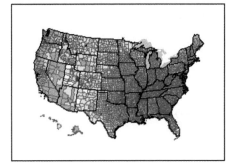

Prepare GIS data for a local health study

In this section you will create a map showing neighborhood "walkability" by adding layers from a variety of sources, in various data formats, and in various projected coordinate systems. You will carry out several steps involving data frame and map layer projections. You will start with several shapefiles obtained from the Pittsburgh City Planning Department, all saved as NAD 1983 Pennsylvania south state plane coordinates. To these layers, you will add data from an ArcInfo interchange file, which you will import into an ArcInfo coverage and then transform into a shapefile. You will also add a CAD from an engineering firm and, finally, an aerial photograph.

Add an ArcView shapefile

1   In ArcMap, click File, New, My Templates, Blank Document, and OK to begin a new map document.

2   Click the Add Data button ✚ , navigate to your **\GistutorialHealth\PAGIS** folder, click **NeighStatePlane.shp**, and click Add.

3   Rename the layer **Neighborhoods**.

4   In the table of contents, right-click the Layers data frame, click Properties, and click the Coordinate System tab.

You can see that the current coordinate system is state plane. The data frame automatically inherits the projection of the first map layer added, if you have not explicitly already set the data frame projection, which is the state plane of Neighborhoods. So, regardless of the projection of additional layers, ArcMap will project them, on-the-fly, to the state plane coordinates of Neighborhoods.

5   Close the Data Frame Properties dialog box and symbolize the map with hollow fill color.

Check the coordinates in the lower right corner of the map to see that they are in feet units, corresponding to state plane.

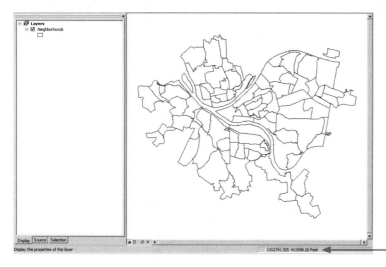

State plane coordinates

6   Save the ArcMap map document as **\GistutorialHealth\Tutorial4-4.mxd**.

YOUR TURN

Add Sidewalks.shp, Parks.shp, and Topo25ft.shp to the map document. Carry out the following tasks for these layers:

- Symbolize these layers so that Sidewalks is a light gray color, Parks is a green color, and Topo25ft is a light tan color.

- Use the Labels tab of the Layer Properties window to turn on labels (using the label features in this layer check box) for Topo25ft with ELEV as the label field. Use a brown font color and use the Placement Properties button to set the properties to Curved and On the line.

- Label Parks using Name. Choose Placement Properties and click the Remove duplicate labels radio button.

The end result is a very jumbled and unusable map, which you will remedy next.

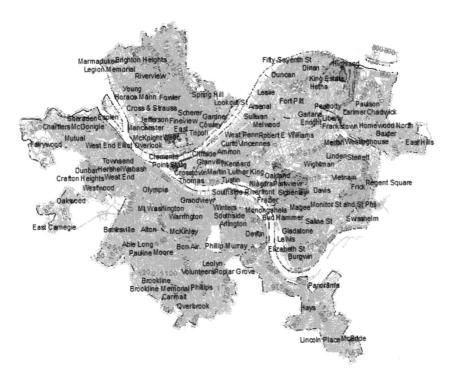

Set scale ranges

Here you will set layers to turn on when zoomed below a scale of 1:24,000, which is a common scale for viewing detailed features of maps. Alternatively, you could zoom to a scale that you find appropriate, read the scale from the Standard toolbar, and use it for scale range properties.

1   **Right-click the Topo25ft layer and click Properties.**

2   **Click the General tab and click the Don't show layer when zoomed radio button.**

3   **In the Out beyond 1 box, type 24000.**

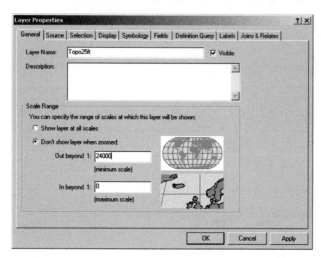

4   **Click OK.**

The topography layer will now not display at the current scale.

5   **Zoom into the map until you are below a scale of 1:24,000.**

Scale below 1:24,000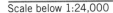

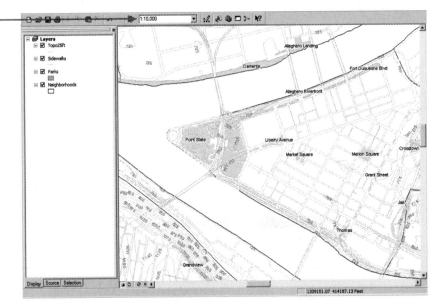

6   **Zoom to the full extent of the map.**

YOUR TURN

Change the scale to turn the sidewalks and parks off when zoomed beyond 1:24,000. Try out your map at exactly 1:24,000 by typing that scale into the scale field on the Standard toolbar and pressing enter.

Add a CAD file

You will next add a CAD file showing Pittsburgh's rivers, which was created by a local engineering firm. CAD map layers often do not have any accompanying data on projections, which is the case with the rivers CAD drawing. This layer, however, has the same state plane projection as Neighborhoods, so it overlays the previously added shapefiles correctly. You will add a spatial reference for rivers, making it capable of being reprojected.

1 **Zoom to the full extent.**

2 **Click the Add Data button** 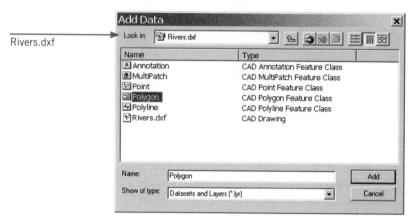 **, navigate to your \GistutorialHealth\PAGIS folder, double-click Rivers.dxf, click Polygon, and click Add. (If necessary, click OK on the warning message.)**

Rivers.dxf

3 **In the table of contents, click the plus (+) sign beside Rivers.dxf Polygon and double-click the symbol for Continuous, 7, 25.**

4 **Symbolize the Rivers.dxf Polygon layer with a light blue fill color.**

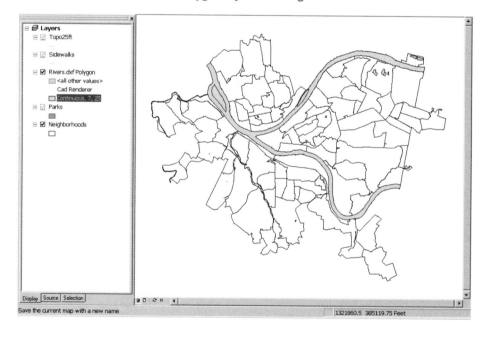

5   Click the ArcCatalog button 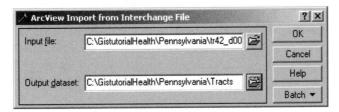 on the Standard toolbar.

6   In the Catalog tree, navigate to **\GistutorialHealth\PAGIS**.

7   In the PAGIS folder, right-click **Rivers.dxf** and click Properties, General, Edit.

8   Under the Coordinate System tab of the Spatial Reference Properties window, click Import. If necessary, navigate to the **\GistutorialHealth\PAGIS** folder, click **NeighStatePlane**, and click Add.

9   Click the Save As button, and browse to the **\GistutorialHealth\PAGIS** folder. In the Save Coordinate System dialog box, type **Rivers** in the Name field, then click Save, OK, OK, and close ArcCatalog.

Rivers now has a correct spatial reference, so in a later step where you change the data frame projection to UTM, it will also reproject correctly.

Import an ArcInfo interchange file and add an ArcInfo coverage

In this section, you will import an ArcInfo interchange file downloaded from the U.S. Census Web site into an ArcInfo coverage (which has geographic coordinates), and export it to a shapefile. While you will not use this layer directly in this tutorial, it has value: for example, you could use it to display the number of school-age children per tract. You are already familiar with symbolizing area maps, so you will skip that step here. The census tract map that you will import is for all of Pennsylvania. In tutorial 7, you will learn how to extract any subset of a map layer, such as for Pittsburgh.

1   Click the ArcCatalog button 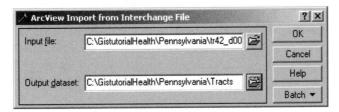 on the Standard toolbar.

2   Click View, Toolbars, ArcView 8X Tools.

3   In the resulting ArcView 8X Tools window, click the Conversion Tools drop-down arrow, then click Import from Interchange File.

4   In the ArcView Import from Interchange File dialog box, click the browse button for the Input file, browse to your **\GistutorialHealth\Pennsylvania** folder, click **tr42_d00.e00**, and click Open.

5   Click the browse button for the Output dataset field, browse to your **\GistutorialHealth \Pennsylvania** folder, name the output **Tracts**, click Save, and click OK.

This step imports the interchange file as an ArcInfo coverage.

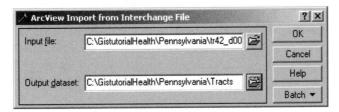

6　**Close ArcCatalog.**

7　**In ArcMap, click the Add Data button.**

8　**Navigate to \GistutorialHealth\Pennsylvania, click Tracts, and click Add.**

9　**Open My Computer, browse to your \GistutorialHealth\Pennsylvania folder, and examine the Tracts and Info folders.**

Each coverage has its own folder, such as Tracts and Info.

10　**Close My Computer.**

Export the coverage to a shapefile

ArcInfo coverages cannot be edited in ArcMap. If you wish to edit coverages, such as the Tracts coverage, you must export them as either a shapefile or geodatabase format. In this case you will export Tracts as a shapefile.

1　**In the table of contents, right-click the tracts polygon coverage, point to Data, and click Export Data. In the Export Data dialog box, make sure the option to use this layer's data source is chosen.**

Tracts is a map layer in the Pennsylvania folder, which might be used for any part of the state. The state plane coordinate system of projections has two projections for Pennsylvania—north and south—so it's best to leave this layer in latitude–longitude coordinates and let ArcMap project it on-the-fly to the data frame's projection.

2　**Click the browse button, navigate to \GistutorialHealth\Pennsylvania and name the output Tracts, click Save, OK, and Yes to add the layer to your map.**

3　**Symbolize Tracts to have no fill color and a blue outline.**

4　**If necessary, turn off the tracts polygon layer in the table of contents.**

Neighborhoods and tracts should be coterminous (share boundary lines), but are not in this case because GIS analysts in Pittsburgh's City Planning Department edited their map layers to align them with aerial photographs. You will remedy this mismatch problem later in tutorial 7.

5　**Right-click Tracts, click Properties, click the Source tab, observe that Tracts has geographic coordinates, and close the Properties window.**

Add an event file

To add a table that has x,y coordinates to your map, the table must contain two fields—one for the x-coordinate and one for the y-coordinate. Here you will add a table that has point coordinates in latitude and longitude for schools in Pennsylvania.

1　**Click the Add Data button** **, navigate to \GistutorialHealth\Pennsylvania, and add the table called PASchools.dbf.**

2 With the Source tab clicked in the table of contents, right-click the PASchools.dbf table and click Open to examine the latitude and longitude attributes.

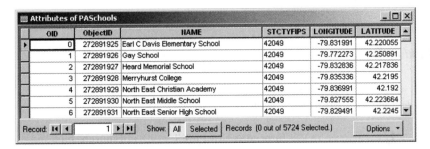

3 Close the attribute table.

4 Right-click the PASchools.dbf table and click Display XY Data.

Next you will add a spatial reference for the event file.

5 In the Display XY Data dialog box, click the Edit button.

6 In the Spatial Reference Properties window, click Select, Geographic Coordinate Systems, North America, North American Datum 1983.prj, and Add.

7 Click the Save As button, browse to the **\Gistutorial\Pennsylvania** folder, type **PASchools** in the Name field, and click Save, OK, and OK.

8 Right-click PASchools Events in the table of contents, click Properties, click the Source tab, observe that the map layer now has a spatial reference, and close the Layer Properties dialog box.

9 Symbolize PASchools Events to have a Square 2 point marker with a purple fill color and symbol size of 7, label its features in the Name field, and define a scale-dependent display for the layer so that it's not visible when zoomed out beyond a scale of 1:24,000.

10 In the table of contents, click the Display tab.

Change the data frame projection to UTM

All map layers have spatial references, so you can change the data frame projection from state plane to another regional projection, such as UTM. When you change the projection and coordinate system of a data frame, ArcMap reprojects all map layers from their current coordinate systems to the one you choose.

1 Right-click Layers in the table of contents, click Properties, then click the Coordinate System tab.

2 In the Select a coordinate system panel, navigate to **Predefined**, **Projected Coordinate Systems**, **UTM**, and **NAD 1983**, click **NAD 1983 UTM Zone 17N**, and click OK. Zoom to a small portion of the map so that all layers are visible.

You will see all layers, which are now in UTM projection and coordinates. Notice at the bottom of your window that coordinates of the UTM are in meters and not feet. In the next step, you will return the data frame projection to state plane.

3   Open the Coordinate System tab of the Data Frame Properties again, navigate to **Predefined**, **Projected Coordinate Systems, State Plane, NAD 1983 (Feet)**, click **NAD StatePlane Pennsylvania South FIPS 3702 (Feet)**, and click OK.

Add an aerial photo to the map

The aerial photo that you will add is in UTM coordinates and has a spatial reference. So, when you add it to the map document and data frame, ArcMap will reproject it on-the-fly to state plane coordinates.

1   Click the Add Data button ![add data icon], navigate to **\GistutorialHealth\PAGIS**, click **pittsburgh_east_pa_ ne.tif**, and click Add.

2   Right-click Pittsburgh_east_pa_ne.tif and click Zoom to Layer.

3   In the table of contents, right-click the image layer, click Properties, and click the General tab.

4   Click the Don't show layer when zoomed radio button, and type **24000** in the Out beyond field.

5   Click the Source tab, scroll down in the property panel, and observe that the image layer has UTM coordinates.

6   Click OK in the Properties window.

7   Click the Find button ![find icon] on the Tools toolbar.

8   In the Find window, type **East Liberty** in the Find box, select Neighborhoods from the In drop-down list, and click the Find button.

9   Right-click East Liberty in the lower panel, click Zoom to, and close the Find window.

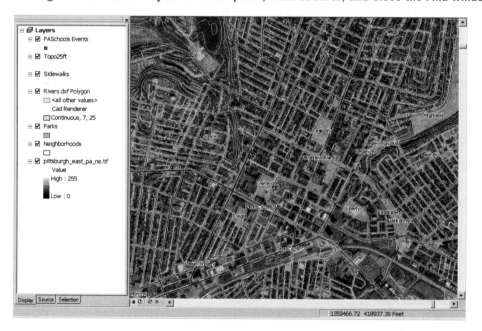

Improve labeling at the neighborhood level

Many of Pittsburgh's public schools are old and the building facilities are not equipped for students to participate in physical activities. The school district task force concerned with child obesity can use your map to identify possible off-campus playgrounds.

1   **Right-click PASchools Events and click Properties, the Labels tab, and the Symbol button.**

2   **In the Symbol Selector dialog box, click the Properties button.**

3   **In the Editor dialog box, click the Mask tab, click the Halo radio button, change the Size to 1, and click the Symbol button.**

4   **Select a light purple fill color and click OK on all the open dialog boxes.**

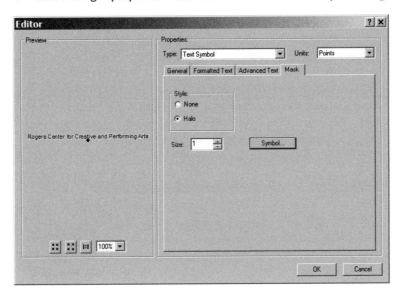

TURN

YOUR

Add a white size-1 halo to the Parks layer labels. Also, give Neighborhoods a blue size-2 halo and label the neighborhoods.

Set parks as semitransparent

1   Right-click any toolbar and click Effects.

2   Click the Layer drop-down arrow and click Parks.

3   Click the Adjust Transparency button.

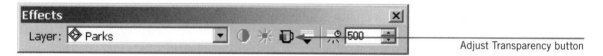

Adjust Transparency button

4   Slide the transparency level to 50%.

5   Close the Effects toolbar.

6   Save your map document.

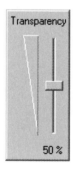

Summary

Small-scale maps (e.g., countries of the world) using disease-related data are best symbolized with size-graduated point markers. The kinds of maps that you made for AIDS prevalence clearly depicted the parts of the world most heavily impacted by this disease. The more familiar alternative, the choropleth map, has distortions and mixed signals caused by variation in the size of polygons. Bigger polygons appear more important than smaller ones, and color value of polygon fill colors is supposed to effectively communicate the perceived meaning.

Large-scale maps for health applications tend to correspond to detailed phenomena and programs, and consequently need detailed maps. You were able to assemble a map document for Pittsburgh, Pennsylvania, and its neighborhoods that allows a GIS analyst working for a child antiobesity task force to identify parks and playground areas near schools that possibly could be used for physical education programs. As is typical of large geographic scale GIS projects, you found that needed GIS layers were available, but from various sources, in various spatial data formats, and in different projections.

You saw that ArcGIS has all of the tools and functions necessary to handle importing, transforming, and projecting practically any map layers of use to you. In addition, you used ArcMap and ArcCatalog to add spatial reference data to map layers and the data frames that hold them, so that ArcMap can project map layers on-the-fly from a mix of projections to a common one for display. ArcGIS has practically any projection available that you would care to use.

In summary, this tutorial has furthered your ability to handle many of the initial problems confronting GIS analysts in real projects. You overcame potential stumbling blocks by adding and properly projecting available spatial data into a map document.

Exercise assignment 4-1

Map showing world infant mortality rates and life expectancy

Problem:

According to the World Health Organization, approximately 10.5 million children under the age of 5 die every year, but great progress has been made since 1970 when this number was 17 million. The highest mortality rates are in developing countries, and almost half of children who die before reaching age 5 live in Africa. A primary cause of these high child mortality rates is the HIV/AIDS epidemic. In this exercise you will create maps showing infant mortality rates similar to the map that you created comparing worldwide AIDS cases. Data was obtained from the U.S. Census International Database (IDB) for the year 2005, and the infant mortality rate is defined as infant deaths per 1,000 live births.

Start with the following:

- **C:\GistutorialHealth\World\InfantMortalityRates**—polygon shapefile of infant mortality rates by country. Note: Zero values indicate no data was available for that country. Field definitions are as follows:
  IM_Male = Infant Mortality Rate Males
  IM_Female = Infant Mortality Rate Females
  LE_Male = Life Expectancy Males
  LE_Female = Life Expectancy Females

- **C:\GistutorialHealth\World\World_30.shp**—graticule lines of constant latitude and longitude at 30° intervals.

Create maps comparing infant mortality rates and life expectancy

Create a new project called C:\GistutorialHealth\Answers\Assignment4\Assignment4-1.mxd that includes a layout comparing four maps showing infant mortality rates by country and life expectancies for males versus females. Use your judgment as to the break points, color, size, title(s), projection, and so forth.

Create a layout for your map and export the map as a PDF file called C:\GistutorialHealth\Answers \Assignment4\Assignment4-1.pdf.

Save your project as C:\GistutorialHealth\Answers\Assignment4\Assignment4-1.mxd.

Exercise assignment 4-2

Map comparing walkable neighborhoods

Problem:

A recent study conducted in San Diego and published in the American Journal of Public Health (September 2003), identified 60 percent obesity rates in low-density, nonwalkable neighborhoods as compared to 35 percent in walkable neighborhoods. The Centers for Disease Control and Prevention (CDC) has determined that obesity is lowest in countries and neighborhoods that allow for significant walking and biking. Many studies are trying to determine what makes a neighborhood more walkable than others. Some reasons might include neighborhood amenities, sidewalk conditions, or safety. An interesting map comparison would include two neighborhoods at the same scale in the same city. In this exercise, you will compare two Pittsburgh neighborhoods. One is a neighborhood with many shops and activities. The other is currently undergoing a revitalization process. In addition to GIS maps, photos of each area are also helpful in the walkability analysis.

Start with the following:

- **C:\GistutorialHealth\PAGIS\NeighStatePlane**—polygon shapefile of Pittsburgh neighborhoods.

- **C:\GistutorialHealth\PAGIS\Buildings**—polygon shapefile of Pittsburgh buildings.

- **C:\GistutorialHealth\PAGIS\StreetsCL**—polyline shapefile of Pittsburgh streets.

- **C:\GistutorialHealth\PAGIS\Sidewalks**—polyline shapefile of Pittsburgh curbs.

- **C:\GistutorialHealth\PAGIS\Walnut.jpg**—photographs of Walnut Street, Shadyside neighborhood, Pittsburgh, Pennsylvania.

- **C:\GistutorialHealth\PAGIS\FifthForbes.jpg**—photographs of Fifth and Forbes Avenue, Central Business District neighborhood, Pittsburgh, Pennsylvania.

Create large-scale neighborhood maps

Create a new project called C:\GistutorialHealth\Answers\Assignment4\Assignment4-2.mxd with a 14 x 8.5 - inch layout containing two data frame maps, both at a scale of 1:2,000. (Note: The map units for this project should be feet.) Include the above layers, symbolized identically, in both data frames.

In one data frame, zoom to the Pittsburgh neighborhood of Shadyside. Select Walnut Street between Aiken and Negley Streets and zoom to these streets at a scale of 1:2,000. Be sure to select a bright, thick color for the selection.

In the second data frame, zoom to the Central Business District neighborhood. Select the streets Fifth and Forbes between Grant and Wood Streets and zoom to these streets at a scale of 1:2,000.

Add the photographs from above to the data frame and other map elements that you think are important.

Export your map as a JPEG file called C:\GistutorialHealth\Answers\Assignment4\Assignment4-2.jpg.

What to turn in:

If you are working in a classroom setting with an instructor, you may be required to submit the exercises you created in chapter 4. Below are the files you are required to turn in. Be sure to use a compression program such as PKZIP or WinZip to include all files as one ZIP document for review and grading. Include your name and assignment number in the ZIP document <YourNameAssignment4.zip>.

ArcMap projects

C:\GistutorialHealth\Answers\Assignment4\Assignment4-1.mxd
C:\GistutorialHealth\Answers\Assignment4\Assignment4-2.mxd

Exported maps

C:\GistutorialHealth\Answers\Assignment4\Assignment4-1.pdf
C:\GistutorialHealth\Answers\Assignment4\Assignment4-2.jpg

OBJECTIVES

Download U.S. Census Bureau TIGER/Line map files
Identify and download data from U.S. Census Bureau Summary File tables
Prepare census tables for use in mapping
Join tabular data to boundary map layers
Create a geodatabase for integration of data
Build a map for analysis of elevated blood levels of lead in children

GIS Tutorial 5

Downloading and preparing spatial data

Health-care scenario

A program manager for the lead hazard program in a county health department wants to create a map to show local pediatricians how lead may be affecting children. He wants a map that shows locations of homes that were built before 1970—when lead was still used in paint—and the number of children with elevated blood levels of lead. He can then focus on problem neighborhoods and set up meetings with physicians in those areas to make them aware of populations that are at risk for lead poisoning. He recommends that such populations be screened more carefully.

Solution approach

As the GIS analyst, you need to work with both internally and externally obtained data for this project. Available in the health department is a sample of residences showing elevated blood levels of lead in children in a table of census tract-level counts of cases. (Tutorial 6 covers the processing steps needed to produce such data from individual records, so you don't have to do this here.) So the internal data is ready and your remaining work focuses on data from external sources. The desired map is easy enough to design and produce, but as is often the case, you will need to do much set-up work, first downloading basemaps and data, and then preparing them for ArcMap.

Many spatial data sources with download facilities are available on the Internet. Two major Web-based sources that can meet many health and other mapping needs are maintained by the U.S. Census Bureau and ESRI. Both Web sites provide major collections of data at no cost.

The U.S. Census data tables are called Summary Files: (a) Summary File 1 (SF1) from the short-form census is compiled from the questions asked of all people and (b) Summary File 3 (SF3) from the long-form census includes sample data based on questions asked of approximately one household in six, covering income, education, occupation, and mode of travel to work.

For the case at hand, the Census Bureau provides in its SF3 collection the needed housing data, namely, the median year that structures were built. Census tracts provide a natural unit of analysis, being homogeneous neighborhoods of around 4,000 people, so you will download both census tract boundaries and the data.

The Census Bureau cannot have the census tabular data already prepared and joined to maps because there are simply too many census variables—over 16,000! Corresponding map files would be too large and cumbersome to use. Instead, you can join selected census tract data with a census tract map's attribute table. Fortunately, ArcMap is able to join two or more data tables if the input tables share a common identifier attribute.

A data table has a specific format and structure. It is rectangular in shape and made up of rows of data (records) that include attributes in columns that are identifiers or characteristics of entities—geographic entities in the case of GIS, such as census tract areas, street centerlines, and so forth. Each column lists data for a single attribute. If viewed in a spreadsheet program, such as Excel, the first row of data contains attribute names, but all additional rows contain only attribute data, with no summary rows such as totals.

At least one attribute must have a unique, non-null identifier value for each row. In database terminology, this is the table's primary key. For example, the composite FIPS code for census tracts is unique across the entire United States and its possessions. This code is a composite of state, county, and tract identifying numbers. An example is 42003010300, where 42 is Pennsylvania's FIPS code, 003 is Allegheny County's FIPS code, and 010300 is a tract's ID. The county FIPS code and tract ID repeat in other states, but as a composite with the state FIPS code, it is unique. You can use the composite FIPS codes for tracts in the lead study.

To get the census mapped, you will follow this approach:

1 Download the data.
2 Clean up the data.
3 Extract map features of interest.
4 Join datasets.
5 Place project datasets in a geodatabase.

With all data preparation work completed, you will create a choropleth map for the housing data by tract and a dot density map layer for elevated blood levels of lead. A dot density map is an alternative to using a choropleth map and uses a random distribution of points within polygons to portray concentrations.

Download spatial and attribute data from the U.S. Census Bureau

From the U.S. Census Bureau's Web site, you can download census-related map layers with unique identifiers for polygons such as census tract IDs, but not census attribute data such as population, age, sex, race, income, and so on. You need to download the census demographic data separately from the Bureau's American FactFinder Web site, perform some data preparation steps on it, and finally join it to the corresponding map layer.

Lower Internet Explorer's security setting for downloading

If you are using Internet Explorer and your Internet security settings are too high, you may not be able to download datasets. A simple solution is to temporarily decrease the Internet security settings so you can download all records simultaneously. Be sure you change these settings before going to the Census Web site. If you are using another Web browser, such as Mozilla Firefox, these steps may be unnecessary.

1   **Launch Internet Explorer or a similar Web browser.**

2   **Click Tools, Internet Options, and the Security tab.**

3   **Click Custom Level.**

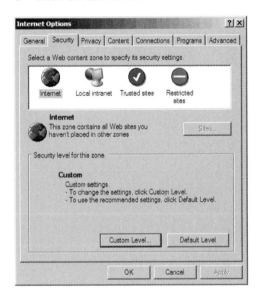

4   **Select Medium-low as the security setting, click Reset, Yes, OK, and OK.**

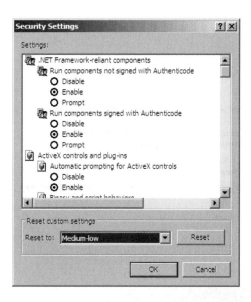

You will now be able to download files successfully. We recommend that you return security to a higher level, such as medium or higher, when you are finished.

Download a TIGER/Line shapefile for census tracts

The end result of these steps is a downloaded copy of the shapefile, tr42_d00.shp. Because Internet sites change often, some of the screen captures below may be different from yours. If you have difficulty downloading the shapefile, we have included it in **\GistutorialHealth\Pennsylvania** as **Copytr42_d00.shp**. If you need to use the copy, use ArcCatalog to delete the word "Copy," changing the name to **tr42_d00.shp**.

1   **From Internet Explorer or another Web browser, open the site www.census.gov.**

2   **Click the TIGER link from the Geography section of the U.S. Census home page.**

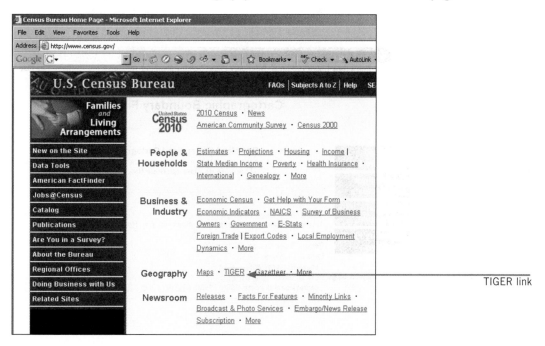

3   On the resulting TIGER page, click the Census Bureau Maps link that is located under the heading TIGER-Related Products.

TIGER®-Related Products

Census Bureau Maps link

- Census Bureau Maps -- Census 2000 Map Series, Online Mapping, and Census 2000 Centers of Population
- Cartographic Boundary Files -- Generalized boundary files in (.shp), (.e00) and (ASCII) formats.
- Census 2000 Block Relationship Files -- 1990 to 2000 Census Blocks.
- Census 2000 Census Tract Relationship Files -- 1990 to 2000 Census Tracts.
- LandView® -- A Federal Geographic Data Viewer
- TIGER/CTSI® -- Census Tract Street Index® Version 4 -- A tool for 1990 HMDA/CRA reporting. **No longer available**

4   Click the Boundary Files link, then, on the resulting Cartographic Boundary Files page, click the Download Boundary Files link.

Download Boundary Files link

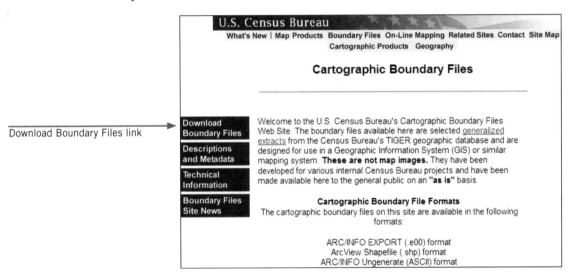

5   Click the Census Tracts 2000 link.

Census Tracts 2000 link

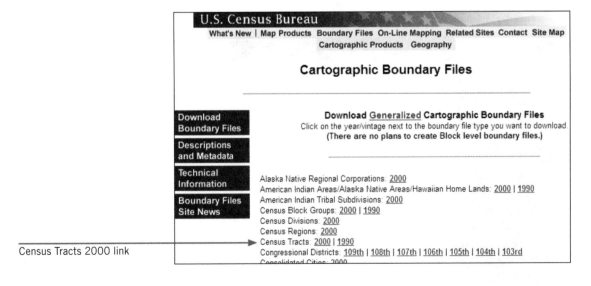

6　Scroll down to the section for downloading shapefile format map layers and click the
　　Pennsylvania - tr42_d00_shp.zip link.

Pennsylvania census
tracts 2000 link

```
Census 2000: Census Tracts
 in ArcView Shapefile (.shp) format

New Jersey - tr34_d00_shp.zip (505,739 bytes)
New Mexico - tr35_d00_shp.zip (358,834 bytes)
New York - tr36_d00_shp.zip (1,301,504 bytes)
North Carolina - tr37_d00_shp.zip (1,208,781 bytes)
North Dakota - tr38_d00_shp.zip (199,526 bytes)
Ohio - tr39_d00_shp.zip (927,851 bytes)
Oklahoma - tr40_d00_shp.zip (596,917 bytes)
Oregon - tr41_d00_shp.zip (646,915 bytes)
Pennsylvania - tr42_d00_shp.zip (1,371,674 bytes)
Rhode Island - tr44_d00_shp.zip (64,204 bytes)
South Carolina - tr45_d00_shp.zip (675,669 bytes)
South Dakota - tr46_d00_shp.zip (236,986 bytes)
Tennessee - tr47_d00_shp.zip (1,056,705 bytes)
Texas - tr48_d00_shp.zip (2,373,016 bytes)
Utah - tr49_d00_shp.zip (356,832 bytes)
Vermont - tr50_d00_shp.zip (86,347 bytes)
Virginia - tr51_d00_shp.zip (990,447 bytes)
Washington - tr53_d00_shp.zip (878,652 bytes)
```

7　Save the file to your **\GistutorialHealth\Pennsylvania** folder and use a compression program to
　　extract **tr42_d00.shp** to the same folder.

YOUR TURN

Launch ArcCatalog, navigate to \GistutorialHealth\Pennsylvania, and select tr42_d00.shp.
Right-click this shapefile, choose properties and the x,y coordinate system tab. Change the
coordinate system to Geographic Coordinate Systems, North American Datum, 1983.

Clean the census tract attribute data

Downloaded, this shapefile does not have a convenient tract identifier that you can use to join to the census tract
data that you will download. So your next step is to create the needed identifier, the complete FIPS number for
each tract. The advantage of the FIPS identifier is that it is unique across counties, so in the future you can work
with a multiple-county region if necessary. In case you have difficulty with this and the next section, we have
provided a copy of the finished product as **Copy_Finished_ tr42_d00.dbf** in the **\GistutorialHealth\Pennsylvania**
folder. Just delete tr42_d00.dbf and change the name of Copy_Finished_tr42_d00.dbf to **tr42_d00.dbf**.

1　**Start ArcMap with a new empty map.**

2　**Click the Add Data button ✚ , navigate to your \GistutorialHealth\Pennsylvania folder, click
　　tr42_d00.shp, and click Add.**

3　**Open the attribute table for the tr42_d00 layer.**

4　**Choose Options, Add Field.**

5   Type **TractNum** as the name, select Double as the type, and click OK.

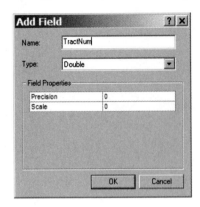

6   Choose Options, Add Field.

7   Type **TractInt** as the name, select Text as the type, and click OK.

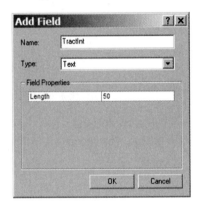

8   Scroll horizontally to the far right-hand side of the table, right-click the TracInt field name, click Field Calculator, and click Yes.

9   Enter [STATE]&[COUNTY]&[TRACT] as the calculation and click OK.

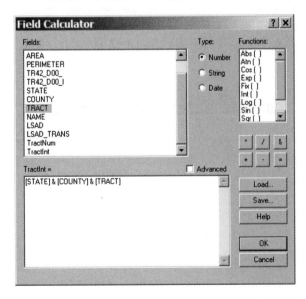

10 Right-click the TractNum field name, click Field Calculator, and click Yes.

11 Erase the expression that you entered in step 9 from the Field Calculator. Click Int( ) in the functions panel, then click TractInt so the calculation appears as Int([TractInt]).

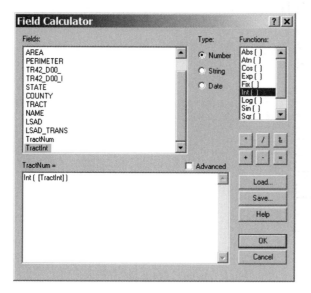

12 Click OK.

13 Right-click the TractNum field, and click Sort Ascending.

14 Select the first 2,282 records.

Note: An easy way to select the first 2,282 records is to scroll to the record that has 9 characters and select that one and all above it.

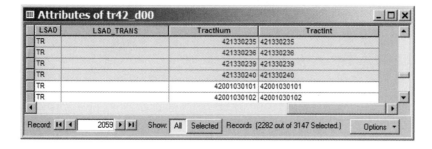

15 Click the Selected button so only the selected records display.

16 Right-click the TractNum field name, click Field Calculator, and click Yes.

17   Enter **[TractNum]*100** as the calculation and click OK.

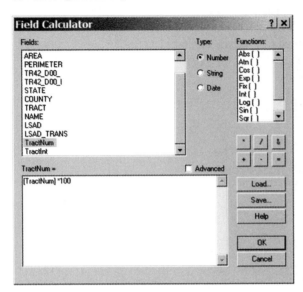

18   Click the All button to show all the records again, then click Options, Clear Selection.

19   Right-click the field name LSAD_TRANS, select Delete Field, and click Yes.

YOUR TURN

Delete fields LSAD, NAME, TRACT, STATE, TR42_D00_, and TR42_D00_I.

Download an SF3 housing variable

Housing data was downloaded from the U.S. Census American FactFinder site. Note that because Internet sites change often, some of the screen captures below may be different from yours. If you have difficulty downloading the file in this section, we have included a backup copy called **Copy_dt_dec_2000_sf3_u_data1.xls** in the **\GistutorialHealth\ACHD** folder.

1   **Using Internet Explorer, go to www.factfinder.census.gov.**

2   **Click Data Sets, Decennial Census in the left panel.**

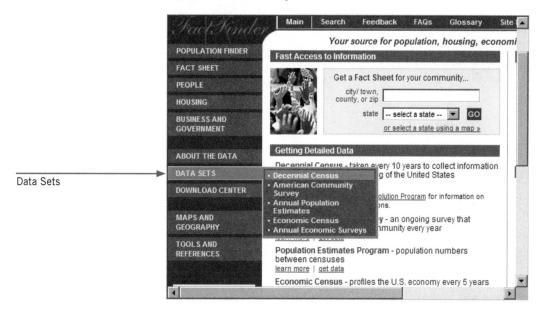

Data Sets

3   **Click the Census 2000 Summary File 3 (SF 3) - Sample Data radio button and click Detailed Tables.**

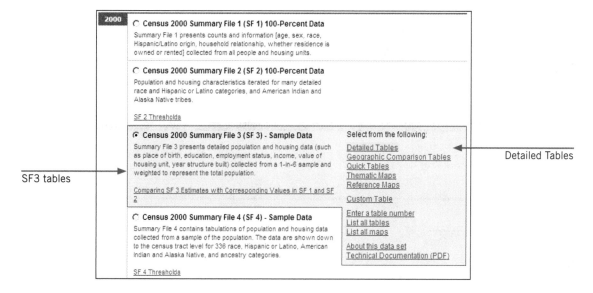

SF3 tables

Detailed Tables

4 **Click Census Tract as the geographic type, Pennsylvania as the state, Allegheny as the county, All Census Tracts, Add, and Next.**

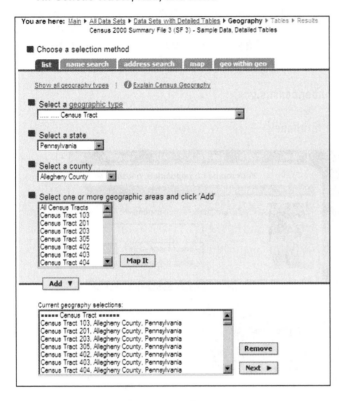

5 **Scroll down and click H35 Median Year Structure Built from the list of tables, then click Add, and Show Result.**

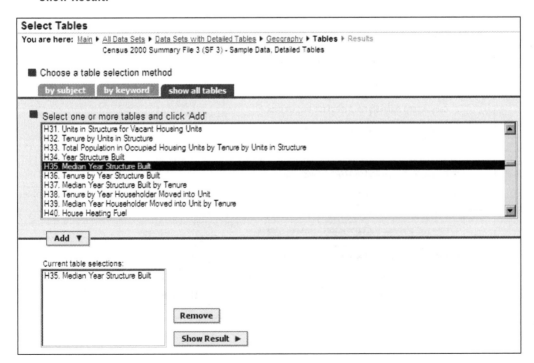

The resultant table shows each census tract and the median year structures were built.

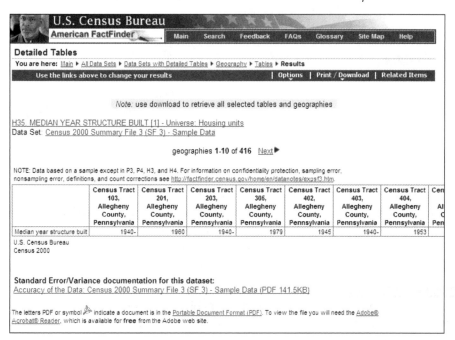

Download census tract housing data from SF3

1   **Click Download from the Print/Download menu.**

2   **Click the Microsoft Excel (.xls) radio button and click OK.**

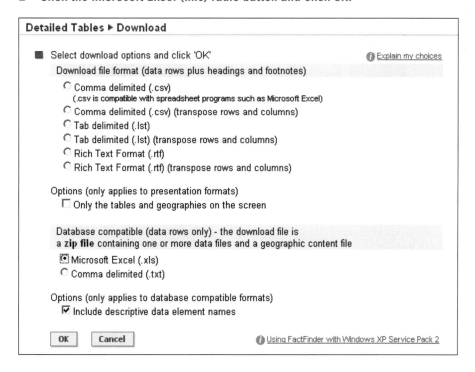

3 Save the files in the **\GistutorialHealth\ACHD** folder with the name given to it by the Census Bureau (output.zip) and extract them to the same folder.

Clean census tract SF3 data in Microsoft Excel

Many downloaded files contain unnecessary text, making them unusable in ArcMap. Here you will do some cleanup in Excel. If you have difficulty in this section, we have provided a copy of the finished product as **Copy_YrBuilt.dbf** in the **\GistutorialHealth\ACHD** folder.

1 Open **dt_dec_2000_sf3_u_data1.xls** in Microsoft Excel.

You should see 418 rows of data in the spreadsheet. If your file does not contain all the census tracts, you probably did not lower your browser Internet settings enough. In addition, you need to clean up this table before it can be joined to the TIGER/Line shapefile. If you are in a situation where you cannot decrease your security level, remember to use the fallback copy of this file that was provided for you (Copy_dt_dec_2000_sf3_u_data1.xls).

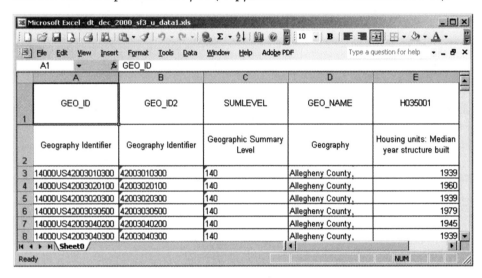

2 Click the row selector button at the start of row 1 and click the Align Left button on the formatting toolbar.

3 Click Format, Row, Height, type **15**, and click OK.

4 Click in cell B1 and type **Tract**.

5 Click in cell E1 and type **YrBuilt**.

6 Click the row selector button for row 2, click the Edit menu, and click Delete.

7 Click the column selector D, click the Edit menu, and click Delete.

8   Similarly delete columns C then A.

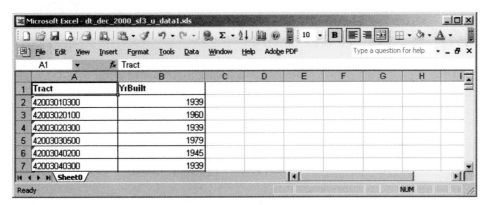

Now you have stripped the table to only the data you need.

9   Click the File menu and click Save As. Change the Save as type to DBF 4 (dBASE IV) (*.dbf), name
the file **YrBuilt**, click Save, Yes, close Excel, and click No.

10   Save your speadsheet as **C:\GistutorialHealth\ACHD\YrBuilt.xls**.

Save file as dBASE using Microsoft Access

1   Launch Microsoft Access.

2   Open **YrBuilt.xls**.

3   Choose the External Data tab.

4   In the Export options, choose the drop-down arrow under More.

5   Export the Excel Spreadsheet as file format DBF 4 (dBASE IV), naming the file **YrBuilt.dbf**.

Note: If you do not have Microsoft Excel or Access, you can get a copy of the YrBuilt.dbf file
in C:\GistutorialHealth\ACHD, called copy_YrBuilt.dbf.

Download a shapefile from the ESRI Census TIGER/Line data Web site

You will download a layer for county municipalities from the ESRI Web site. This will help the director of the lead program identify what municipalities or neighborhoods have the most cases. Note that because Internet sites change often, some of the screen captures below may be different from yours. If you have difficulty downloading these files, we have included the zipped shapefiles **copy_ccd0042003.zip, copy_lkB42003.zip**, and **copy_wat42003.zip** in the **\GistutorialHealth\ACHD** folder as a backup.

Download spatial data

1   Launch a Web browser and go to **www.esri.com/data/resources/geographic-data.html**.

A list of data portals, including *geographynetwork.com, geodata.gov,* and other resources are listed here.

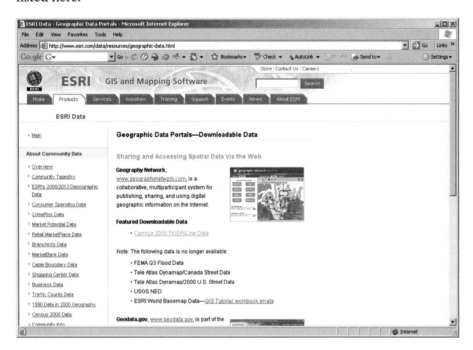

2   Click Census 2000 TIGER/Line Data.

3   Click Preview and Download from the side menu.

4   Click PA on the map.

5   Select Allegheny as the county and click the Submit Selection button.

6   Click the check boxes for County Census Divisions 2000, Line Feature—Rails, and Water Polygons.

7   Scroll to the bottom of the page and click the Proceed to Download button.

8   Click Download File and download the contents to your **\GistutorialHealth\ACHD** folder.

9   Use a compression program and extract the shapefiles you just downloaded—**tgr42003ccd00.shp**, **tgr42003wat.shp**, and **tgr42003lkB.shp**—to the **\GistutorialHealth\ACHD** folder. Be sure to extract all associated files (i.e., .shp, .shx, and .dbf).

YOUR TURN

Add the spatial reference North American Datum, 1983, to each of these shapefiles.

Build a map layer for elevated blood levels of lead in children

Several data and map preparation steps remain before you can produce the desired map. You have to extract tract polygons for Allegheny County from the larger Pennsylvania shapefile of tracts. Next you need to join the prepared SF3 data to the Allegheny County census tract map.

Extract Allegheny County tracts from Pennsylvania tracts

1   If necessary, start ArcMap with a new empty map.

2   Click the Add Data button ![add data], browse to your **\GistutorialHealth\Pennsylvania** folder, and add **tr42_d00.shp**.

This action adds all of Pennsylvania's census tracts.

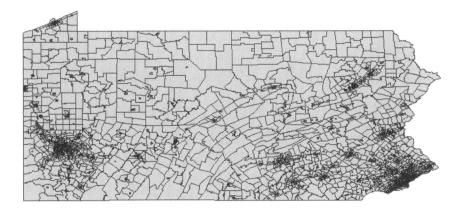

3   Click the Selection menu and click Select By Attributes.

4   In the list of fields, double-click "COUNTY", click the = button, then, in the expression box, type '003' just after the equals sign (be sure to include the single quotes around the value).

This action builds an expression to choose census tracts in Allegheny County, Pennsylvania, whose county code is 003.

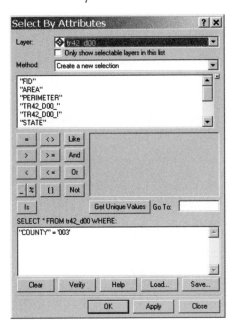

5   Click OK.

Only Allegheny County tracts are selected.

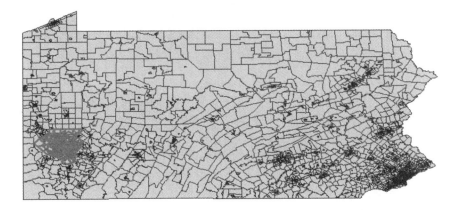

6   In the table of contents, right-click tr42_d00, click Data and Export Data.

7   In the Export Data window, click the data frame radio button, browse to your **\GistutorialHealth\ACHD** folder, name the output **Tract003**, click Save, OK, and Yes.

8   Right-click tr42_d00 and click Remove.

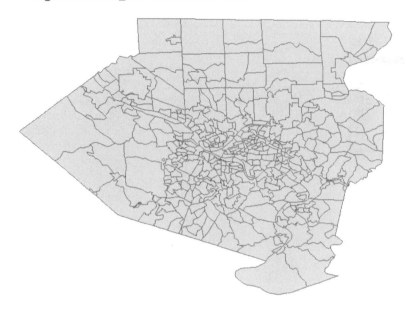

Create a text data type version of the Tract ID

At the beginning of this tutorial, you downloaded some SF3 data that included the tract FIPS code as a text field, which you saved as the attribute Tract in YrBuilt.dbf. You also went to great lengths to create the same tract FIPS number, now in the Tract003.dbf attribute table. That version of the tract FIPS number has a numeric data type. Soon you will need to join YrBuilt.dbf to Tract003.dbf so you can map the YrBuilt attribute based on common values of tract FIPS numbers in both tables. The join function, however, will only work when you join fields of the same data type, so here you will make a text field and use it to store the values currently in the TractNum field in Tract003.dbf.

1   In the table of contents, right-click Tract003 and select Open Attribute Table.

2   In the Attributes of Tract003 table, click the Options button and click Add Field.

3   In the Add Field window, type **Tract_1** in the Name field, change the Type to Text, change the field length from 50 to **11**, and click OK.

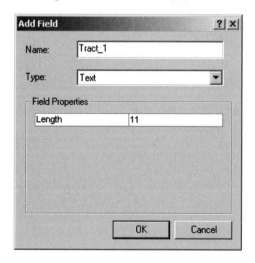

4 In the Attributes of Tract003 table, locate and right-click the Tract_1 field name, click Field Calculator, and click Yes.

5 In the Field Calculator window, double-click TRACTNUM and click OK.

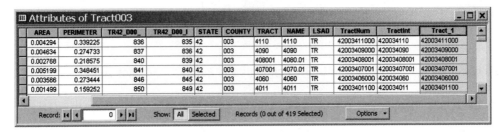

AREA	PERIMETER	TR42_D00_	TR42_D00_I	STATE	COUNTY	TRACT	NAME	LSAD	TractNum	TractInt	Tract_1
0.004294	0.339225	836	835	42	003	4110	4110	TR	42003411000	420034110	42003411000
0.004634	0.274733	837	836	42	003	4090	4090	TR	42003409000	420034090	42003409000
0.002768	0.218575	840	839	42	003	408001	4080.01	TR	42003408001	42003408001	42003408001
0.005199	0.348451	841	840	42	003	407001	4070.01	TR	42003407001	42003407001	42003407001
0.003586	0.273444	846	845	42	003	4060	4060	TR	42003406000	420034060	42003406000
0.001499	0.159252	850	849	42	003	4011	4011	TR	42003401100	420034011	42003401100

Record: 0   Show: All Selected   Records (0 out of 419 Selected)   Options ▾

6 Close the Attributes of Tract003 table.

Join housing and elevated blood cases tables to census tract map

Here you will join the housing data to the census tract's attribute table using the census tract field common to both tables.

1   In the table of contents, right-click Tract003, click Joins and Relates, and click Join.

2   In step 1 of the Join window, select Tract_1 from the drop-down list.

3   In step 2, browse to your \GistutorialHealth\ACDH folder, click YrBuilt.dbf, and click Add.

4   In step 3, select TRACT from the drop-down list.

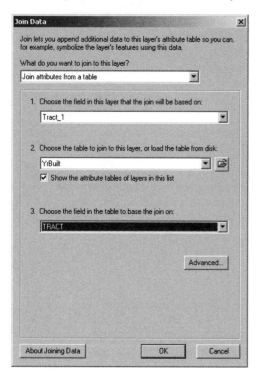

5   Click OK and Yes.

6   Open the attribute table for Tract003 and scroll to the right.

Fields from the Attributes of the YrBuilt table are now joined to the Attributes of Tract003 table and the field names are now prefixed with names of their source table.

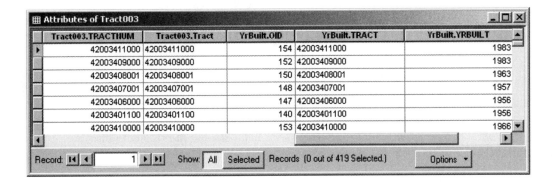

YOUR TURN

Join ElevatedBloodCases.dbf, found in your \GistutorialHealth\ACHD folder, to Tract003.shp. Use the Tract003.Tract_1 field in step 1 of the Join dialog box and the TRACT field in step 3 of the dialog box.

Permanently join tables

To permanently join these tables, you will export the joined layer as a new shapefile. The resulting shapefile will have all attributes in the joined tables as permanent attributes.

1   In the table of contents, right-click Tract003 and click Data, Export Data.

2   Save the output to your **\GistutorialHealth\ACHD** folder and name it **MedianYrHousing.shp,** but do not add the exported data to your map.

3   Remove Tract003 from your map.

Create a new personal geodatabase

1 Close ArcMap without saving.

2 Launch ArcCatalog.

3 Expand the catalog tree in the left panel, if necessary, and click the **ACHD** folder under the **\GistutorialHealth** folder.

4 Click the File menu.

5 Click New, then click Personal Geodatabase.

6 Type **LeadStudy.mdb** as the geodatabase name.

Import a shapefile into the geodatabase

1 Right-click **LeadStudy.mdb**, click Import, and then click Feature Class (single).

2 For the Input Features, click the browse button, navigate to **\GistutorialHealth\ACHD**, click **MedianYrHousing.shp**, then click Add.

3 Type **MedianYrHousing** as the Output Feature Class Name.

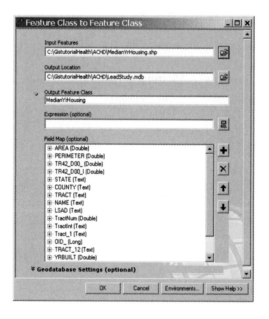

4 Click OK and Close once the import is complete.

YOUR TURN

From your \GistutorialHealth\ACHD folder, import tgr42003ccd00.shp as Municipalities, tgr42003wat.shp as Rivers, and tgr42003lkB.shp as Railroads. When you are finished, close ArcCatalog.

Build a lead-study comparison map

Now that you have downloaded and prepared the spatial and attribute data, you are ready to build a map using this data.

Add map layers and project the data frame

1   Start ArcMap with a new empty map.

2   Click the Add data button, browse to your **\GistutorialHealth\ACHD** folder, and double-click **LeadStudy.mdb**.

3   In the Add Data dialog box, hold down the Ctrl key, click the MedianYrHousing, Rivers, and Municipalities feature classes (leave railroads out), then click Add.

4   Add another copy of MedianYrHousing.

5   Project the data frame using the following selections in Coordinate System properties: Predefined, Projected Coordinate Systems, State Plane NAD 1983 (Feet), NAD_1983_StatePlane_ Pennsylvania_South_FIPS_3702_Feet.

6   Save the project as **Tutorial5-1.mxd** in your **\GistutorialHealth\ACHD** folder.

Symbolize map layers

1   Move Rivers to the top of the table of contents and symbolize it with a light blue fill color.

2   Move Municipalities second from the top and symbolize it with hollow fill color and a black outline with a width of 1.5.

3   Right-click the top copy of MedianYrHousing, click Properties, the Symbology tab, Quantities, and Dot density.

4   In the Field Selection frame, click ELEVBLOODL, and click the arrow button (>) to transfer that column to the main frame.

5   Double-click the symbol marker in the right panel and change its color to red, then click OK.

6   In the background panel, click the line symbol button [   ] and change the color to No Color.

7   Change the dot size to 1.5 and the dot value to 1, and click OK.

A dot value of 1 means that there is one randomly placed dot in a tract for every case that occurred in the tract.

8   Symbolize the second copy of MedianYrHousing as a choropleth map using the field YRBUILT with three classes and manual break points of 1950, 1960, and 1970.

9　Use a gray color ramp and reverse it so that the highest color value is for the oldest category of median year built. (To reverse the color ramp, click the first symbol in the list and select Flip symbols.)

10　Double-click each of the three symbols and change the Outline Color to No Color.

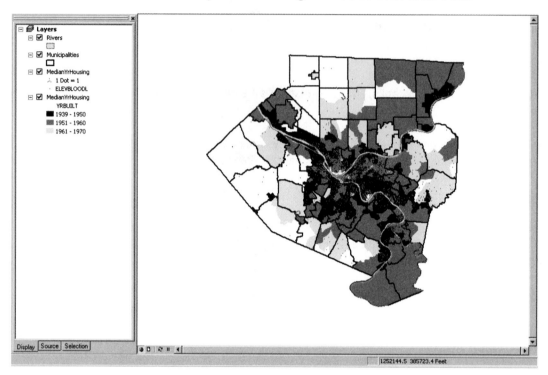

As expected, you can see a correlation between houses built before 1970 and cases of elevated blood levels of lead in children. Probably other factors affect the frequency of elevated lead levels. Because of our familiarity with Pittsburgh, we can see from the patterns in the dot density layer that poverty is also at work here. You will pursue this possibility in an exercise in which you download data on poverty and add it to the tract layer for display and analysis.

11　Save your map document as **Tutorial5-1.mxd** in your **\GistutorialHealth** folder and exit ArcMap.

Summary

Preparing data to do analytic work, including GIS-based studies, requires multiple skills and almost always takes more time than anticipated. This tutorial focused on skills that you need for obtaining external data—from the U.S. Census Bureau and ESRI Web sites, in this case—and getting them into the right form for use in ArcMap. You had to find and download needed census data, fix several problems with data values to make them useful, and ultimately join them to a tract map layer. Then, using skills learned in tutorials 3 and 4, producing the map itself took relatively few steps.

In regard to substantive knowledge gained, you provided evidence that the built environment affects children's health. Parts of Allegheny County built before 1970 tend to have concentrations of cases with elevated lead levels in children's blood. The exercises in this tutorial asked you to add additional census variables to the map in an attempt to further explain this variable.

Next, in tutorial 6, you will prepare internal data for use in GIS. If internal records contain street addresses or geocodes such as ZIP Codes or county IDs, then you can spatially enable them to become map features.

Exercise assignment 5-1

Map housing values compared to elevated blood levels of lead

Problem:

Tutorial 5 mapped locations of children with elevated blood levels of lead. The map clearly showed that cases were clustered in Pittsburgh neighborhoods with older houses and also in neighborhoods with high poverty, low educational attainment, and other low socioeconomic status indicators. Some studies show that financial housing statistics are a better indicator of the economic status of a city than poverty rates. In this exercise, you will download U.S. Census data that provides median housing values and median and gross rents. This data can be downloaded from the U.S. Census Web site and added to the childhood lead study.

Start with the following:

- **U.S. Census SF3 Geographic Comparison Data Table (GCT-H9. Financial Housing Characteristics: 2000) downloaded from**
  - http://factfinder.census.gov/
  - Data Sets, Decennial Census
  - Census 2000 Summary File 3 (SF 3) - Sample Data
  - Geographic Comparison table for Allegheny County, Pennsylvania

Note: If you have trouble downloading this data, two files with housing data for Allegheny County can be found in **C:\GistutorialHealth\ACHD\Exercise5-1_CensusHousingData.zip**.

- **C:\GistutorialHealth\ACHD\MedianYrHousing.shp**—Allegheny County census tracts extracted from Pennsylvania census tracts in tutorial 5 and joined with housing and elevated blood data.

Note: This file can also be found in C:\GistutorialHealth\SolutionsComparisons\Chapter5\LeadStudy.mdb. You will need to export it from the Leadstudy personal geodatabase in order to import it to a new one that you will create in the exercise.

Create comparison maps for financial housing data and elevated blood levels

Edit the downloaded data of financial housing characteristics so it can be joined to the shapefile MedianYrHousing. You will import this file to the personal geodatabase below.

Create a new geodatabase called C:\GistutorialHealth\Answers\Assignment5\ACHD.mdb with the above files (including new housing values) imported into it.

Create a new project called C:\GistutorialHealth\Answers\Assignment5\Assignment5-1.mxd that includes a map comparing housing variables, median housing values, *or* median gross rent that you downloaded from the census Web site and the number of elevated blood levels of lead in each census tract. Use your judgment as to the break points, color, size, title(s), and so on.

Export the map as a PDF file called C:\Gistutorial\Health\Answers\Assignment5\Assignment5-1.pdf.

EXERCISES

Exercise assignment 5-2

Map housing complaints compared to elevated blood levels of lead

Problem:

The local health department investigates complaints from landlords and tenants about unsafe or unsanitary housing conditions. This data can also be mapped and compared to locations showing elevated blood levels. In this exercise, you will create a map of housing complaints by census tract and compare this to the elevated blood levels.

Start with the following:

- **C:\GistutorialHealth\ACHD\MedianYrHousing.shp**—Allegheny County census tracts extracted from Pennsylvania census tracts in tutorial 5 and joined with housing and elevated lead levels data.

Note: This file can also be found in C:\GistutorialHealth\SolutionComponents\Chapter5\Leadstudy.mdb.

- **C:\GistutorialHealth\ACHD\HousingComplaints.dbf**—database providing the number of housing complaints by census tract in Allegheny County, Pennsylvania.

Create comparison maps for housing complaints and elevated blood levels

Import the above files into C:\GistutorialHealth\Answers\Assignment5\ACHD.mdb. Please note that if you already completed assignment 5-1, the MedianYrHousing shapefile will already be imported into the geodatabase.

Create a new project called C:\GistutorialHealth\Answers\Assignment5\Assignment5-2.mxd that includes a map comparing housing complaints and the number of elevated blood levels in each census tract. Use your judgment for the break points, color, size, title(s), and so forth.

Export your map as a JPEG file called C:\GistutorialHealth\Answers\Assignment5\Assignment5-2.jpg.

What to turn in:

If you are working in a classroom setting with an instructor, you may be required to submit the exercises you created in chapter 5. Below are the files you are required to turn in. Be sure to use a compression program such as PKZIP or WinZip to include all files as one ZIP document for review and grading. Include your name and assignment number in the ZIP document <YourNameAssignment5.zip>.

Geodatabase

C:\GistutorialHealth\Answers\Assignment5\ACHD.mdb with imported files

ArcMap projects

C:\GistutorialHealth\Answers\Assignment5\Assignment5-1.mxd
C:\GistutorialHealth\Answers\Assignment5\Assignment5-2.mxd

Exported maps

C:\Gistutorial\Health\Answers\Assignment5\Assignment5-1.pdf
C:\Gistutorial\Health\Answers\Assignment5\Assignment5-2.jpg

EXERCISES

OBJECTIVES

Create new health-care map layers using internal and local data

Geocode ZIP Code data

Spatially join and aggregate point data to create choropleth maps

Batch geocoded address data

Interactively rematch address data to fix input errors

GIS Tutorial 6

Geocoding tabular data

Health-care scenario

Top management at a major hospital in Pittsburgh, Pennsylvania, has recently hired you as a GIS analyst. You have downloaded basemaps and data from the U.S. Census Bureau and ESRI Web site to use as GIS data. Now you need to spatially enable some of the hospital's internal data, using ArcMap geocoding features. Patient data used in this tutorial is fictional data created by the book's authors.

One of your future projects is to evaluate alternative locations for a satellite hospital clinic. You will create two new layers to make a good starting point for this endeavor. You will have two datasets: (1) all other hospitals in the county, and (2) a multistate sample of patient data. You will need to locate the hospitals as precisely as possible to assess the local competition. Your own hospital, however, will have a number of specialties with no local competitors, so you will need to visualize patient demand patterns not only locally but also in the multistate area. For this purpose, you will not plot individual residential locations of patients. Instead, counts of patients by ZIP Code will best meet your needs.

Solution approach

The most common form of geocoding uses sophisticated programs to match tabular street address data with street address attributes in a line map layer of streets. Such programs use "fuzzy matching" to account for variations in abbreviations and spellings of address data, just as your postal delivery person does when getting the mail to you.

TIGER/Line street files, available from the U.S. Census Bureau, are limited. They do not have data and separate points for every street address, such as 33 Pine Ave. Instead, each TIGER/Line feature is a block-long street segment with street numbers for only the beginning and end of the block on both odd and even sides of the street. For Pine Ave., the data might be street numbers 1, 2, 99, and 98 if the street has blocks broken up by hundreds in house numbers. The ArcMap geocoding program for TIGER/Line-formatted streets finds the relevant street segment for a street address and approximates a point location using simple interpolation of starting and ending street numbers and points.

Geocoding is not always successful; for example, the input address data in a tabular file may have errors, or the TIGER/Line street map may be missing streets or attribute data. ArcMap, when geocoding addresses, provides a report giving the number of matched addresses, resulting in points on the map, and unmatched addresses. Often it is possible to improve the match rate by using the ArcMap interactive rematching interface and making corrections, record by record.

Typically, you can expect about an 85 percent match rate, without rematching, in urban areas with good input data. The range of successfully matched addresses, however, is quite high, typically from 50 percent to 99 percent, depending on both the quality of the input address data and street maps used. Street maps from commercial vendors generally provide better address match rates than the free TIGER/Line maps.

On your map, the competitor hospitals need to be located as points, so you plan to geocode hospital data to a street network. The number of hospitals is relatively few, so the manual steps following automated geocoding that will correct nonmatching addresses will not be very time consuming. Your goal is to geocode all of the hospitals.

In some cases, you will not need or even want very fine detail, such as when estimating demand patterns and protecting privacy of data as in this tutorial. In such cases, geocoding to ZIP Code polygons may be sufficient. Generally, tabular ZIP Code data is accurate, so you can expect match rates in the 90 percentile, placing points at ZIP Code centroids. While you could geocode patient residences to the street network, you decide that ZIP Code counts of patients will be sufficiently fine-grained for studying location patterns, especially over a tristate region.

Geocode patients to ZIP Code centroids

Suppose you have a table containing the addresses of the patients and their ZIP Codes. Using the ArcMap geocoding program, you can create a point layer from the ZIP Code list. The point features use the centers, or centroids, of ZIP Code polygons. The data you will use in this section contains fictitious ZIP Code locations, analogous to actual locations, for individual patients in a hospital.

Begin a new health-care map project

1   **Start ArcMap with a new empty map.**

Add a ZIP Code layer

First you will geocode the health-care organization's database of patients by ZIP Code for a ZIP Code map of the entire United States. You will then do a more detailed site selection analysis of the region where most patients are clustered.

1   **Click the Add Data button** ➕ **, navigate to C:\GistutorialHealth\UnitedStates, click ZipCodes.shp, and click Add.**

That action adds the ZIP Code shapefile for the entire United States.

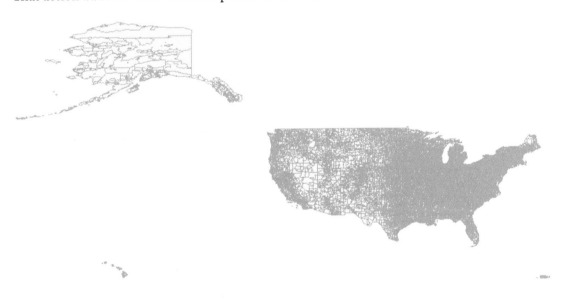

Add patient database and open its attribute table

The input data is Patients.dbf. You will geocode this to a reference layer, ZIP Code polygons. For now, open the input table and observe its attributes.

1   **Click the Add Data button** ➕ **, navigate to C:\GistutorialHealth\SiteSelection, and click Patients.dbf.**

2   In the table of contents, right-click Patients.dbf and click Open.

The table lists ZIP Codes for each patient.

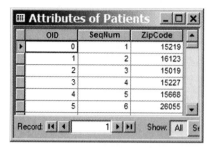

3   Close the table.

Build address locator for ZIP Codes

Before you can geocode the patient locations, you must tell the software which data is the reference data (ZIP Code polygons) and define a set of parameters for how it reads the input data (Patients.dbf). This is done by creating an address locator, which is a stored set of specifications for carrying out the process. After you create and store an address locator, you can reuse it in other geocoding projects.

1   Click the ArcCatalog button.

2   In the catalog tree, navigate to **GistutorialHealth\SiteSelection**.

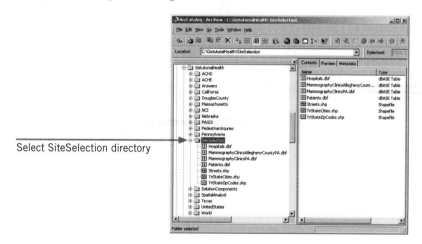

Select SiteSelection directory

3   Click the File menu, click New, and Address Locator.

4   In the Create New Address Locator dialog box, scroll down the list of address locator styles, locate, then click ZIP 5Digit and click OK.

There are many different address locators for different types of reference data.

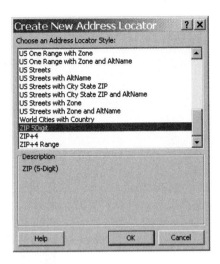

After you click OK, the New ZIP 5Digit Address Locator dialog box opens, allowing you to define the properties of this locator style.

5 Name the new address locator **USAZipCodes**.

6 Within the Primary table tab, click the browse button, navigate to **C:\GistutorialHealth \UnitedStates** and click **ZipCodes.shp**, then click Add.

7 In the Output Fields frame (located in the lower right corner of the dialog box), check the X and Y coordinates box.

You can adjust several settings in the address locator dialog box to affect the outcome of the matched ZIP Codes. The ZIP field in the reference data is automatically located by the setup dialog box and is seen in the Input Address Fields section. Including x,y coordinates in the attribute table is an option, making the resultant data useful in other application software.

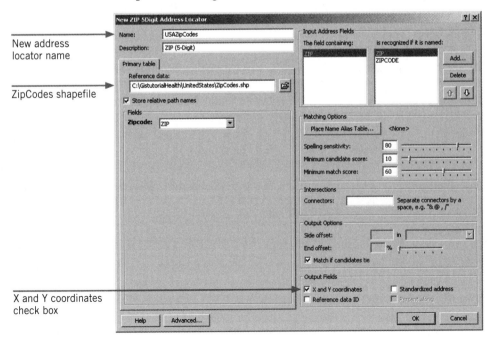

New address locator name

ZipCodes shapefile

X and Y coordinates check box

8   Click OK.

ArcCatalog creates a new ZIP Code address locator in the \GistutorialHealth\SiteSelection folder. You can double-click to open the properties of this locator and change them at any time.

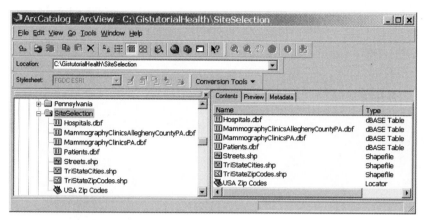

9   Close ArcCatalog.

Add address locator in ArcMap

Now that you have determined the input and reference data and have created an address locator, you are ready to geocode the patients to ZIP Code polygons. First, you must add the address locator in ArcMap.

1   In ArcMap, click the Tools menu, Geocoding, Address Locator Manager, and Add.

2   Navigate to \GistutorialHealth\SiteSelection.

3   Click USAZipCodes, Add, and Close.

Geocode patients using new address locator

1   Right-click Patients.dbf in the table of contents, then click Geocode Addresses and OK.

2   In the Address Input Fields frame, select ZipCode from the ZIP drop-down list.

3   Name the output shapefile **GeocodedPatients.shp** and save it in your **\GistutorialHealth \SiteSelection** folder.

Using the patients table as the input, the address locator will read the values in the ZipCode field and will place points in the corresponding ZIP Code polygons in the reference data. ArcMap will write the output as a new shapefile named GeocodedPatients.shp.

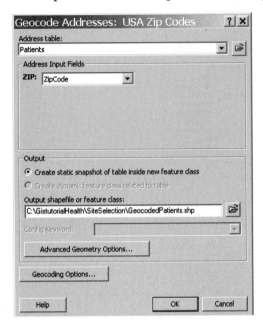

4   Click OK.

ArcMap will process the patient ZIP Codes to the ZIP Code polygons and a results dialog box will appear. The Statistics frame within this dialog box reports how successfully the input data was geocoded. You should have 94 percent (8,739) of the ZIP Codes match, which is good, but it should be possible to get even higher match rates. Records that did not match likely contained incorrect ZIP Code values, or could not find matching records in the ZipCodes shapefile.

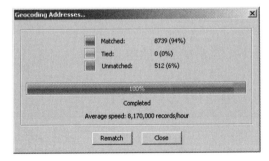

5   Click Close and zoom to the boundary of the 48 contiguous U.S. states. In the table of contents, rename the Geocoding Result: GeocodedPatients layer **GeocodedPatients**.

Points appear in the center of ZIP Codes where patients are located across the United States. Notice that some patients travel quite a distance to the hospital in Pittsburgh. Because hospital administrators are focusing on a new regional site, you will focus on patients in western Pennsylvania only.

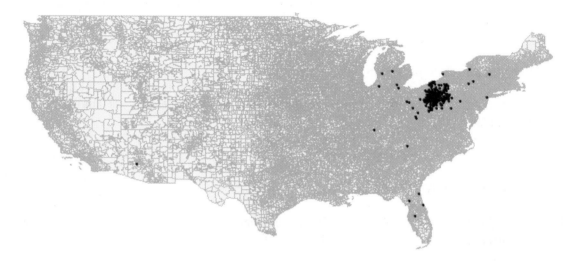

Spatially join patient and ZIP Code layers

A map that shows ZIP Code centroids is misleading because several patients could be at the same point, yet the points do not indicate that. A better way to visualize patients is to create a graduated point-marker or choropleth map that displays the number of patients in each ZIP Code. To enable such a map, you can count patients by ZIP Code using a process known as a spatial join. Here you will spatially join the patient points to ZIP Codes in Ohio, Pennsylvania, and West Virginia only. This will give hospital administrators a good idea of location patterns for regional patients.

Spatially join points to polygons

1   Click the Add Data button ⊕ , navigate to **\GistutorialHealth\SiteSelection**, and add **TriStateZipCodes.shp**.

2   Remove the ZIPCodes layer from the map.

3   Zoom to the TriStateZIPCodes layer.

4   Click the Add Data button again. Add the **\GistutorialHealth\UnitedStates\States.shp** layer to your map. Symbolize the layer with a hollow fill and an outline size of 1.5.

5   At the bottom of the table of contents, click the Display tab.

Notice that the patient locations are mostly in western Pennsylvania but some also exist in Ohio and West Virginia.

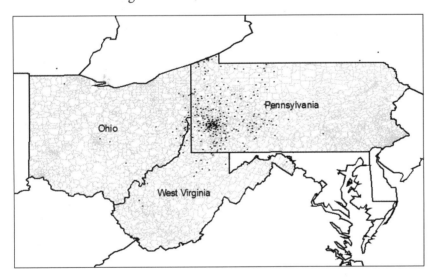

6   In the table of contents, right-click the TriStateZipCodes layer, click Joins and Relates, and click Join.

7   Click the What do you want to join to this layer? drop-down arrow and choose Join data from another layer based on spatial location.

8   **For step 1 of the Join Data dialog box, choose GeocodedPatients from the drop-down list.**

9   **Accept the default settings for step 2. For step 3, name the output TriStatePatients.shp and save it in your \GistutorialHealth\SiteSelection folder.**

10   **Click OK.**

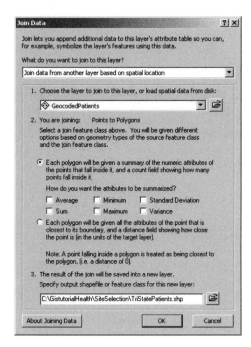

The output is a new polygon shapefile containing ZIP Code boundaries attributed with the patient data.

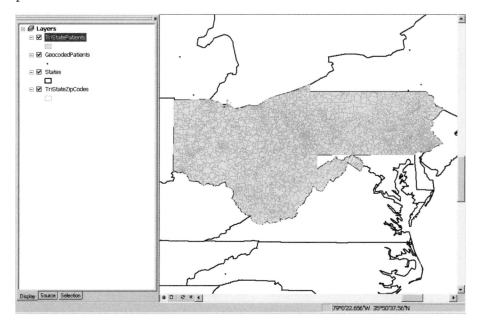

11 Open the attribute table of TriStatePatients and note that ArcMap added a count field with the number of patients in each ZIP Code.

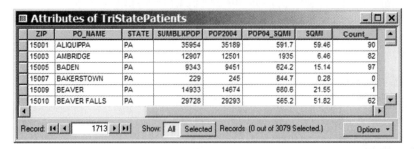

12 Close the attribute table.

Create a choropleth map showing patient counts by ZIP Codes

You can now create a choropleth map based on the patient counts in each ZIP Code.

1   **Turn off the GeocodedPatients and TriStateZipCodes layers.**

2   **Right-click the new TriStatePatients layer and click Properties.**

3   **Click the Symbology tab, choose Quantities, Graduated Colors, and Count_ as the field value.**

4   **Set the break values to 20, 40, 60, and 80. Leave the last break value as 99.**

5   **Change the labels and color ramp to your liking and click OK on the Layer Properties dialog box.**

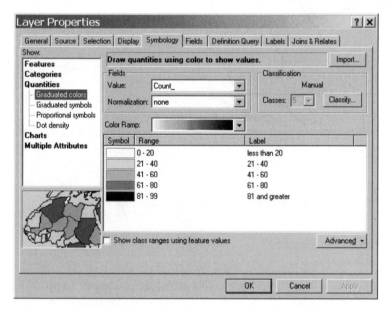

6   **Add the \GistutorialHealth\UnitedStates\Counties.shp layer to your map. Symbolize the layer with a hollow fill and an outline size of 1.15.**

7   **Zoom to southwestern Pennsylvania as shown below.**

You can now see where most of the health-care organization's patients are clustered.

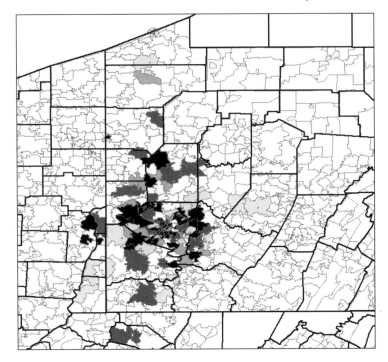

YOUR TURN

Remove the layers TriStateZipCodes and GeocodedPatients. Add and symbolize two additional layers:

\GistutorialHealth\SiteSelection\TriStateCities.shp
\GistutorialHealth\UnitedStates\Interstates.shp

Label the counties with a nice halo label. Save the project as GistutorialHealth\Tutorial6-1.mxd. Based on the resulting map, in what city would you recommend opening a satellite clinic?

Geocode hospital addresses to streets for competitive analysis

Here you will address match the locations of existing hospitals to Allegheny County's streets. The streets used here are Census 2000 TIGER/Line street centerlines downloaded from the ESRI Web site. The ESRI StreetMap data product, which comes with ArcView, is another good resource for street centerlines, especially if you are geocoding across multiple counties or states.

Begin a new health-care map

1   **Start ArcMap with a new empty map. If ArcMap is already open, click the New Map File button on the Standard toolbar.**

Add streets layer

This is the reference layer you will match hospital addresses to.

1   **Click the Add Data button ⊕ , navigate to \GistutorialHealth\SiteSelection, and double-click Streets.shp.**

This action adds the street centerline shapefile for Allegheny County with Pennsylvania south state plane coordinates. This map layer has over 80,000 block-long street segments!

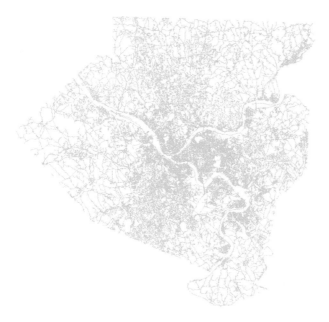

2   **Zoom to the center of the map.**

3 Using the Identify tool, click a line segment, and note fields in each line segment.

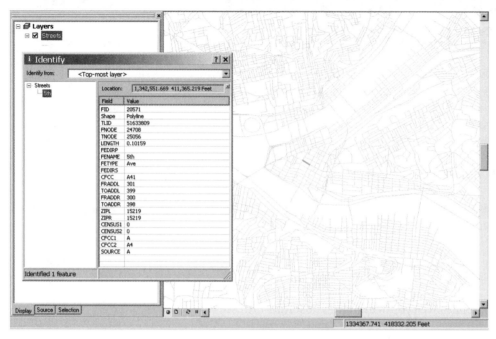

4 Close the Identify window.

Add hospital database

This is the input database that you will use to create point features for each hospital address.

1 Click the Add Data button ✚, browse to **\GistutorialHealth\SiteSelection**, and double-click **Hospitals.dbf**.

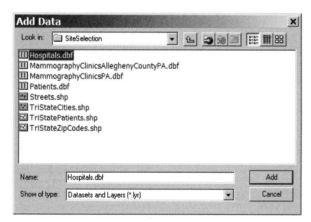

2 In the table of contents, right-click Hospitals.dbf and click Open.

The table lists hospital names, street addresses, ZIP Codes, and the number of beds for each hospital. The address locator will use the ADDRESS and ZIPCODE fields to geocode each record.

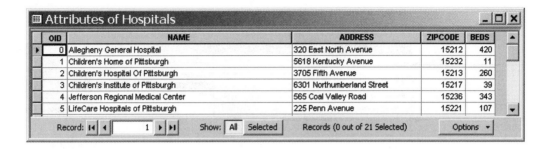

3 Close the Attributes of Hospitals table.

Build an address locator for streets

The steps used to set up the address locator for streets are the same as the ones used in the previous task for ZIP Codes, but some of the parameters will differ because you are geocoding to the street level.

1 Click the ArcCatalog button.

2 In the catalog tree, navigate to **\GistutorialHealth\SiteSelection**.

3 Click the File menu, New, Address Locator, click US Streets with Zone, and click OK.

This choice is necessary because your input file includes street addresses and ZIP Codes (zones). Zones are necessary to break ties due to street names that repeat from one municipality to another.

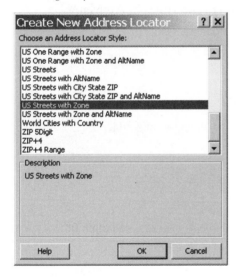

4 Name the new address locator **AlleghenyCountyStreets**.

5 In the Primary table tab, click the browse button, navigate to **\GistutorialHealth\SiteSelection**, and double-click **Streets.shp**.

6 In the Matching Options frame, change the Minimum match score to 65.

7   Check the X and Y coordinates box in the Output Fields frame.

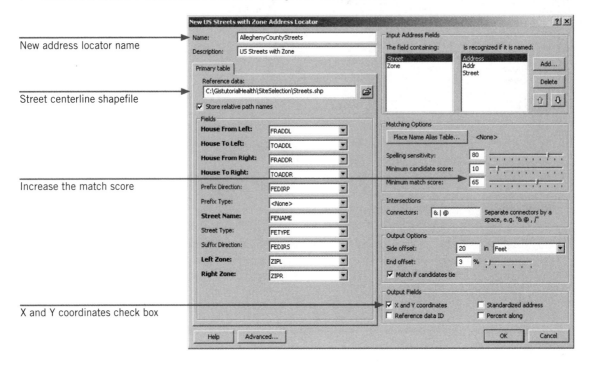

New address locator name

Street centerline shapefile

Increase the match score

X and Y coordinates check box

8   Click OK.

ArcMap creates a new street address locator that is saved in the \GistutorialHealthSiteSelection folder. You will use this locator to geocode hospitals to street centerlines in ArcMap.

9   Close ArcCatalog.

Geocode hospitals using new address locator

1   In ArcMap, click the Tools menu, Geocoding, Address Locator Manager, and Add.

2   Navigate to **\GistutorialHealth\SiteSelection**.

3   Click AlleghenyCountyStreets, Add, and Close.

4   In the table of contents, right-click Hospitals.dbf, click Geocode Addresses, and click OK.

5   From the Street or Intersection drop-down list, choose ADDRESS.

6   From the Zone drop-down list, choose ZIPCODE.

7   Name the output shapefile **GeocodedHospitals.shp** and save it in your **\GistutorialHealth \SiteSelection** folder.

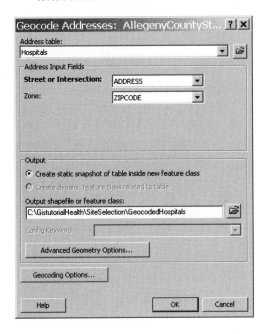

8   **Click OK.**

You should have 76 percent (16) matched, 0 percent tied, and 24 percent (5) unmatched. In the next section you will investigate why some addresses did not match.

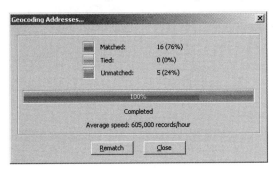

9   **Click Close.**

10 Zoom to the full extent of the map.

Matched points will appear offset 20 feet along the street centerlines where hospitals are located in Allegheny County.

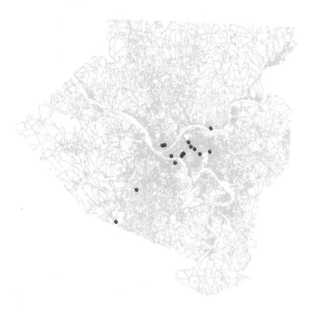

11 Open the attribute table of the matched addresses and note that ArcMap created a number of new fields during the geocoding process.

In the status field, you will see an "M" in the status field if the address is matched, and a "U" if the address is unmatched.

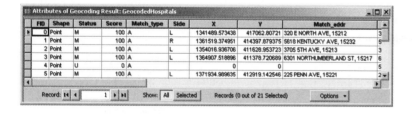

12 Close the table.

Interactively rematch an address

Unmatched records stem from errors in either the reference data or the input data. You need to do some cleanup work in order to match records that didn't match. This is common to the geocoding process. In batch mode, you change the settings of the Address Locator then rerun the process. Another approach is to use an interactive rematch interface where you examine and fix unmatched records case by case. In this section you will use the latter.

1   Click the Tools menu, click Geocoding, Review/Rematch Addresses, Geocoding Result: GeocodedHospitals.

2   The top of the Interactive Rematch dialog box contains a table of unmatched records. In this table, click the record selector button on the left end of the record that contains the value 1401 BLVD OF THE ALLIES (FID 7).

This address has two problems that resulted in a match score of just 51. The first is that BLVD OF THE ALLIES is the street name but the geocoding program thinks that BLVD should be a prefix. Also, the BLVD OF THE ALLIES spans two ZIP Codes: 15219 and 15213. The data has the incorrect ZIP Code. The Interactive Rematch dialog box allows you to examine and repair these types of errors so that you can geocode the unmatched addresses with a better score.

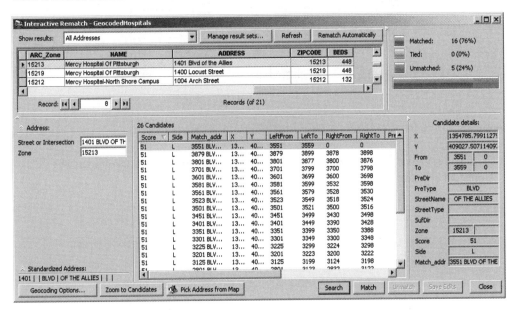

3   In the Street or Intersection box type **1401 BLVD OF THE ALLIES**.

4   In the Zone box type **15219** and press Enter.

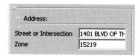

As you make these settings, keep your eye on the Score field in the table of unmatched records. Once you apply the changes, the value for the selected record will change to 100, indicating that a perfect match was made.

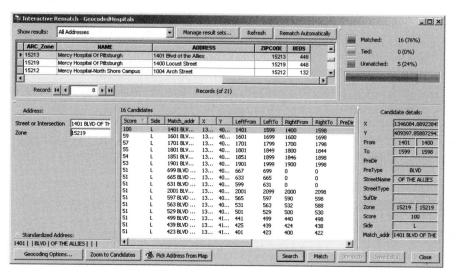

5   Click the Match button located in the lower right corner of the dialog box.

ArcMap changes the status of the record to M (matched), the score to 100, and adds the X and Y coordinates of the address location.

Interactively rematch more addresses

1   In the table of unmatched records, select the record containing 9100 Babcock Boulevard by clicking the gray record selector button that's just to the left of the record.

This record has an incorrect ZIP Code. The correct ZIP Code is 15101.

2   In the Zone box located below the table, change the current value to **15101**, and then press Enter.

Upon entering the new value, many possible candidates appear in the list that's on the lower portion of the dialog box. One has a score value of 100.

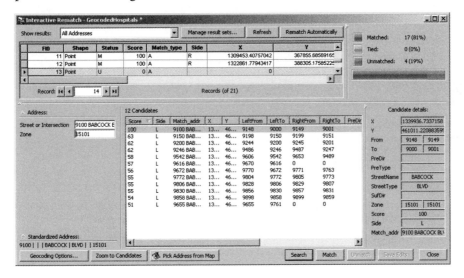

3   In the list of candidates, click the candidate with a score of 100, then click Match.

4   Select the next unmatched record containing 3850 OHara St.

ArcMap shows a 64 percent match score, which is good enough for our purposes.

5   Click Match.

6   Click Close.

The last two addresses are a bit more challenging. For Coal Valley and Delafield Roads you will look at the map to see the problems and find solutions.

7   In the Review/Rematch Addresses dialog box, click Done.

Use street TIGER/Line maps to find addresses

In the previous task you rematched a record that had an error in the input table (hospitals database). Sometimes errors are in the reference tables (street centerlines). For example, TIGER/Line files may be missing values in the address range fields. If you don't see an obvious solution while rematching, or if you are unfamiliar with the geographic region, you may need to look at the street map to help decide what changes are needed. In this section, one of the streets is missing the from and to ranges for a street segment. You will edit the street centerline table to correct this.

1   Click the Selection menu and click Select By Attributes.

2   Click Streets from the Layer drop-down list.

3   In the list of fields, double-click "FENAME", click the = button, press the spacebar on the keyboard, and type 'Coal Valley'.

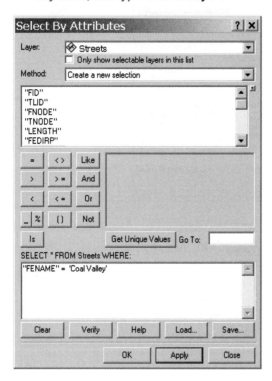

4   Click OK.

You will see Coal Valley selected in the southern portion of the map. The address you are looking for is 565 Coal Valley Road.

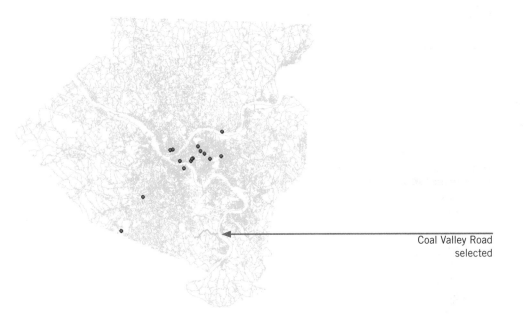

Coal Valley Road
selected

5   Open the Attributes of Streets.

6   In the Attributes of Streets, click the Selected button.

7   Scroll to the right of the table and notice the street ranges for Coal Valley Road.

Notice that many of the streets' from and to ranges are missing.

Missing from
and to ranges

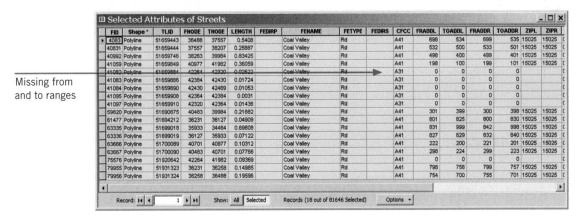

FID	Shape*	TLID	FNODE	TNODE	LENGTH	FEDIRP	FENAME	FETYPE	FEDIRS	CFCC	FRADDL	TOADDL	FRADDR	TOADDR	ZIPL	ZIPR	
4083	Polyline	51659443	36488	37557	0.5408		Coal Valley	Rd		A41	698	534	699	535	15025	15025	
40831	Polyline	51659444	37557	38207	0.25887		Coal Valley	Rd		A41	532	500	533	501	15025	15025	
40992	Polyline	51659748	38263	39964	0.83425		Coal Valley	Rd		A41	498	400	499	401	15025	15025	
41059	Polyline	51659849	40977	41982	0.36059		Coal Valley	Rd		A41	198	100	199	101	15025	15025	
41082	Polyline	51659884	42264	42320	0.02532		Coal Valley	Rd		A31	0	0	0	0			
41083	Polyline	51659886	42384	42430	0.01724		Coal Valley	Rd		A31	0	0	0	0			
41084	Polyline	51659890	42430	42469	0.01053		Coal Valley	Rd		A31	0	0	0	0			
41095	Polyline	51659908	42364	42384	0.0031		Coal Valley	Rd		A31	0	0	0	0			
41097	Polyline	51659910	42320	42364	0.01436		Coal Valley	Rd		A31	0	0	0	0			
59820	Polyline	51690875	40483	39964	0.21682		Coal Valley	Rd		A41	301	399	300	398	15025	15025	
61477	Polyline	51694212	36231	36127	0.04909		Coal Valley	Rd		A41	801	825	800	830	15025	15025	
63335	Polyline	51699018	35933	34464	0.69808		Coal Valley	Rd		A41	831	999	842	998	15025	15025	
63336	Polyline	51699019	36127	35933	0.07122		Coal Valley	Rd		A41	827	829	832	840	15025	15025	
63666	Polyline	51700089	40701	40977	0.10312		Coal Valley	Rd		A41	222	200	221	201	15025	15025	
63667	Polyline	51700090	40483	40701	0.07766		Coal Valley	Rd		A41	298	224	299	223	15025	15025	
75576	Polyline	51920642	42264	41982	0.09369		Coal Valley	Rd		A41	0	0	0	0			
79955	Polyline	51931323	36231	36258	0.14985		Coal Valley	Rd		A41	798	756	799	757	15025	15025	
79956	Polyline	51931324	36258	36488	0.19596		Coal Valley	Rd		A41	754	700	755	701	15025	15025	

Record: 1   Show: All Selected   Records (18 out of 81646 Selected)   Options

8   Close the Attributes of Streets.

9   Zoom to the selected Coal Valley Road features on the map.

10 Use the Identify tool to identify the records of the selected streets.

After exploring the selected street segments, it is apparent that the range between 698 and 699 and 534 and 535 is the closest address range, and the ZIP Code should be 15025.

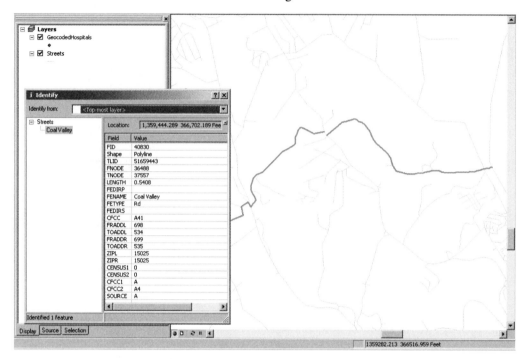

YOUR TURN

Use Select by Attributes to find FENAME=Delafield. Because you do not know the street address number, find a street segment that is closest to the intersection of Delafield and State Route 28 and note the from and to addresses. Note the ZIP Code for Delafield Road and clear the selected features.

Rematch addresses

1   Click the Tools menu and click Geocoding, Review/Rematch Addresses, Geocoding Results: GeocodedHospitals.

2   Click the Match Interactively button.

3   Click the gray record selector for 565 COAL VALLEY ROAD.

4   In the Zone box below the table, delete the existing ZIP Code and press enter.

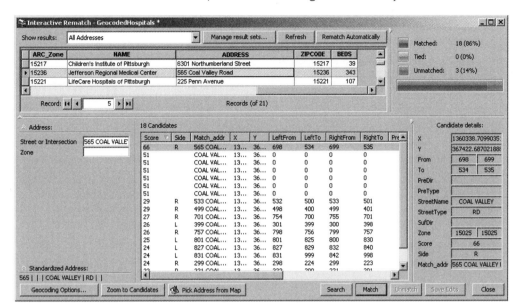

5   Make sure candidate with a score of 66 is selected, then click Match.

6   Click the gray record selector for Delafield Road.

7   In the Street or Intersection box, type **600** before the existing street address, then type **15215** in the Zone box, press Enter when the cursor appears in the ZIP Code box, then press Enter again.

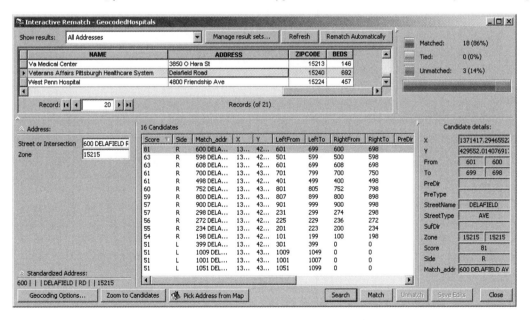

8 Select the Candidate with the score of 81, and click Match then Close.

9 Zoom to the full extent of the data.

10 Save your map as **GistutorialHealth\Tutorial6-2.mxd**.

Congratulations! You successfully geocoded all of the hospitals in your study.

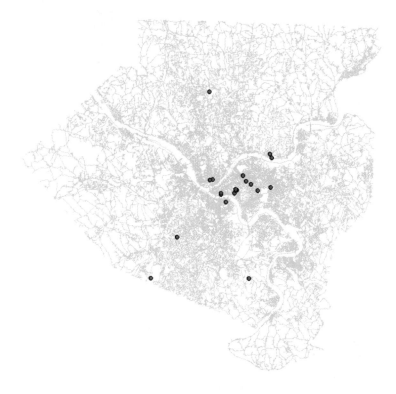

Create a final comparison map

Now that you have patients and hospitals geocoded, you can create a map comparing both layers. An interesting map might compare the hospital locations and number of beds for each hospital (an attribute in the hospital table) to the location of existing patients.

1   **Turn off the Streets layer in the map.**

2   **Click the Add data button and browse to \GistutorialHealth\SiteSelection to add TriStatePatients.shp to your map, symbolized as a choropleth map.**

3   **Navigate to \GistutorialHealth\UnitedStates and add Counties.shp to your map. Symbolize this layer with a hollow fill and label counties with a nice halo label.**

4   **Create a graduated point-marker map showing the number of beds for the existing hospitals compared to a choropleth map of patient locations.**

Can you tell from this map what areas are underserving their current patients and where the health-care organization may want to open a clinic?

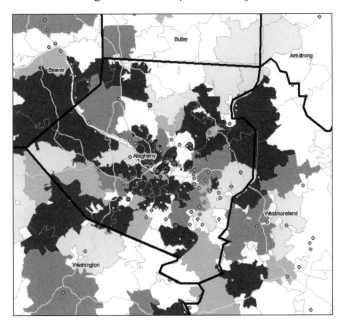

Summary

GIS is useful to the hospital now that you have placed your own patient data and competitor hospitals on the map. Already you can see some promising areas for locating a satellite clinic, either in the northwest or eastern portions of the county.

You have just performed some remarkable feats with GIS by using powerful ArcGIS programs with some of the U.S. map's infrastructure—TIGER/Line street maps and ZIP Code maps. ArcGIS geocoding programs have built-in expertise to accomplish something akin to what your postal delivery person does when interpreting address data relative to actual locations. ArcGIS spatial joins have the unique capability to assign area identifiers to individual points. Then it is easy to aggregate data by spatial identifiers to produce frequencies and other statistics. Geocoding and spatial aggregation are two of the main tasks needed for spatially enabling an organization's data.

Exercise assignment 6-1

Map mammography clinics by ZIP Code compared to females ages 40–64

Problem:

Many health-care organizations are concerned that high malpractice costs, inadequate government and private insurance payments for mammography services, aging screening equipment, a shortage of mammography technicians and radiologists, and the closure of money-losing radiology clinics are among the problems that contribute to high breast cancer rates.

In this exercise, you will geocode mammography clinics in Pennsylvania to ZIP Codes, then compare this to the number of women between the ages of 40 and 64 to see if any areas in the state are inadequately covered. Clinic locations used in this assignment are ones inspected by the federal government, with data downloaded from the FDA Web site, *www.accessdata.fda.gov/scripts/cdrh/cfdocs/cfmqsa/mqsa.cfm.*

Start with the following:

- **C:\GistutorialHealth\SiteSelection\MammographyClinicsPA.dbf**—database of mammography clinic locations in Pennsylvania.

- **C:\GistutorialHealth\Pennsylvania\PAZipCodes.shp**—polygon shapefile of Pennsylvania ZIP Codes.

- **C:\GistutorialHealth\Pennsylvania\PACounties.shp**—polygon shapefile of Pennsylvania counties.

- **C:\GistutorialHealth\Pennsylvania\PATractsFemale40-64.shp**—polygon shapefile of Pennsylvania census tracts with female population between 40 and 64 years old.

Create a map comparing state geocoded mammography clinics to female population

Create a new address locator in C:\GistutorialHealth\Answers\Assignment6 called PAZips that uses style ZIP(5-Digit) and the PAZipCodes shapefile from above.

Begin a new project called C:\GistutorialHealth\Answers\Assignment6\Assignment6-1.mxd that includes a map layout comparing the number of mammography clinics in Pennsylvania ZIP Codes as graduated points and a choropleth map showing the number of females between the ages of 40 and 64.

Hint:

You will need to spatially join geocoded clinics to PAZIPCodes to create a count of the number of clinics shown as graduated points. Set the background color for your points to "No Color."

Save new shapefiles to C:\GistutorialHealth\Answers\Assignment6.

Export your map to a PDF file called **C:\GistutorialHealth\Answers\Assignment6\Assignment6-1.pdf**.

Question:

Create a Word document called **C:\GistutorialHealth\Answers\Assignment6\Assignment6-1.doc** and answer the following questions:

1. Are there areas or counties in the state where it appears that females are not adequately served for mammography screening?

2. What other map layers could you add for a more detailed analysis?

Exercise assignment 6-2

Map mammography clinics in a county by street address

Problem:

In exercise 6-1 you geocoded mammography clinics in Pennsylvania by ZIP Code to investigate the overall supply and demand for mammography clinics. When zoomed in further to a relatively small area within the state, you can see detailed spatial information, with clinics located on the street network. Then, with additional analysis on the population of women, you can start identifying possible relocation areas for existing clinics or locations for new clinics. In this exercise, you will geocode mammography clinics in Allegheny County, Pennsylvania, by street address and compare the resulting spatial distribution of clinics with the population of women by census tract.

Start with the following:

- **C:\GistutorialHealth\SiteSelection\MammographyClinicsAlleghenyCountyPA.dbf**—database of mammography clinic locations in Allegheny County, Pennsylvania.

- **C:\GistutorialHealth\SiteSelection\Streets.shp**—polyline shapefile of Allegheny County streets.

- **C:\GistutorialHealth\Pennsylvania\PACounties.shp**—polygon shapefile of Pennsylvania counties.

- **C:\GistutorialHealth\Pennsylvania\PATractsFemale40-64.shp**—polygon shapefile of Pennsylvania census tracts with female population between the ages of 40 and 64.

Create a map comparing county geocoded mammography clinics to female population

Create a new address locator in C:\GistutorialHealth\Answers\Assignment6 called Allegheny County Streets that uses style US Streets with Zone and the streets shapefile from above.

Create a new project called C:\GistutorialHealth\Answers\Assignment6\Assignment6-2.mxd that includes a map layout showing existing mammography clinics in Allegheny County as a pin map (points) compared to a choropleth map of the female population between the ages of 40 and 64 in the county. To do this, you will need to geocode clinic locations to Allegheny County streets.

Save new shapefiles in **C:\GistutorialHealth\Answers\Assignment6**.

Hint:

ArcMap will not be able to map all clinics. For a variety of reasons, some of the mammography clinics do not match; for example, addresses may have missing street numbers, wrong ZIP Codes, misspellings, or simply be outside of the county. Try using map layers from above, Internet sites such as the U.S. Postal Service, or online mapping programs to find reasons why addresses did not match. Rematch as many unmatched clinics as possible using interactive rematching. Keep a log of the steps you took to rematch and turn this in with your

EXERCISES

assignment as C:\GistutorialHealth\Answers\Assignment6\Assignment6-2.doc. For each address investigated, list the original address, the problem information, source, and correction.

Export the map as a JPEG file called **C:\GistutorialHealth\Answers\Assignment6\Assignment6-2.jpg**.

What to turn in:
If you are working in a classroom setting with an instructor, you may be required to submit the exercises you created in chapter 6. Below are the files you are required to turn in. Be sure to use a compression program such as PKZIP or WinZip to include all files as one ZIP document for review and grading. Include your name and assignment number in the ZIP document <YourNameAssignment6.zip>.

ArcMap projects
C:\GistutorialHealth\Answers\Assignment6\Assignment6-1.mxd
C:\GistutorialHealth\Answers\Assignment6\Assignment6-2.mxd

New shapefiles
C:\GistutorialHealth\Answers\Assignment6\GeocodedMammographyClinicsPA.shp
C:\GistutorialHealth\Answers\Assignment6\GeocodedMammographyClinicsAlleghenyCountyPA.shp
C:\GistutorialHealth\Answers\Assignment6\MammographyClinicsByPAZip.shp

Word document
C:\GistutorialHealth\Answers\Assignment6\Assignment6-1.doc
C:\GistutorialHealth\Answers\Assignment6\Assignment6-2.doc

Exported maps
C:\GistutorialHealth\Answers\Assignment6\Assignment6-1.pdf
C:\GistutorialHealth\Answers\Assignment6\Assignment6-2.jpg

Extract features to build a study area
Dissolve polygons to create neighborhood population counts
Append map layers
Use spatial joins to aggregate data
Create buffers to conduct proximity analysis

GIS Tutorial 7

Preparing and analyzing spatial data

Health-care scenario

Doctors and researchers at a pediatric hospital in Pittsburgh want to explore possibilities for a prevention program to reduce youth pedestrian injuries from cars. They have two hypotheses. One is that poverty contributes to youth pedestrian injuries because of congested and low-quality public spaces for play, resulting in children playing on or near streets. Poverty also leads to a tendency for low parental guardianship, especially in female-headed households. A second hypothesis is that proximity to parks reduces child pedestrian injuries because play areas in parks tend to be away from vehicular traffic, and adults often accompany children to parks and their supervision can prevent accidents. Contrary to the second hypothesis is the possibility of *increased* risk for pedestrian injuries while walking to and from the parks, but researchers believe that the net effect is lowered risks for children living near parks.

One policy-related restriction, peculiar to Pittsburgh, is that any injury-prevention program needs to be designed at the neighborhood level. Pittsburgh has strong neighborhood organizations that would be instrumental for successful implementation. Note that Pittsburgh's neighborhoods are made up of one or more census tracts each, so it should be easy to aggregate census data to the neighborhood level to investigate pedestrian injuries using census data on poverty.

The primary dataset you will use in this study is a collection of 94 cases of severe pedestrian injuries of children up to age 14, drawn from a recent five-year period. The data has several limitations. While we wish that there were no child pedestrian injuries, a sample size of 94 is too few cases from which to draw strong conclusions. For example, Pittsburgh has 90 neighborhoods, so the average is slightly less than one injury per neighborhood, suggesting that there may not be enough data to observe any patterns. In this case, however, youth pedestrian injuries are concentrated in relatively few neighborhoods, so there are patterns to observe and attempt to explain. More observations, however, would make the patterns more reliable.

A second and perhaps more serious limitation is that the data does not include accident addresses, but only the residence addresses of the accident victims. Most youth pedestrian injuries, however, occur near home, so the residence address is a rough location for injury locations. Of course, some accidents occur away from home, for example, near schools. Analysis at the neighborhood level helps reduce the location problem of this data for studying a demographic variable such as poverty, because Pittsburgh neighborhoods are relatively large and self-contained communities with their own primary schools. For studying the effect of parks on reducing youth pedestrian accidents, however, it's more important to have actual accident locations. For example, a child living near a park may be injured near school or someplace relatively distant from home, and the residence data will give incorrect information by associating the accident with the park. However, this error only introduces noise, but no specific patterns or biases, into the study of parks' effect on reducing accidents in their vicinity. If we find any patterns, such as reduced injuries near parks per 10,000 youths, we can assume that the patterns would only be stronger with better location data.

The last limitation is that the injury data is from the only pediatric hospital in Pittsburgh. Serious pediatric injuries may have been treated at other hospitals, but these should be relatively few in number because of the special competencies of the pediatric hospital. Mitigating the problem further is the fact that the pediatric hospital is centrally located in Pittsburgh, and no part of Pittsburgh is more than six miles from the hospital. While the data may be somewhat incomplete, this should not be a serious problem. In any event, it is clear from all of the data limitations that this study is highly exploratory.

Solution approach

In this tutorial you will build an analysis from basemap layers and several data sources, then use GIS in conducting sophisticated spatial analyses. The tasks for building the analysis are many and are fairly comprehensive in the kinds of GIS preparation work that you are likely to encounter. You carried out some of this kind of work in earlier tutorials—there is a lot to remember and some repetition here in new circumstances helps.

The GIS data you will use includes the following:

- Several TIGER/Line map layers in latitude-longitude coordinates for Allegheny County, which includes the city of Pittsburgh, downloaded from the ESRI Web site in tutorial 5
- Two injury datasets that were address matched using TIGER/Line streets by the methods outlined in tutorial 6
- A data table of Summary File 3 (SF3) census data from the Census Bureau Web site used in tutorial 5, which we prepared to yield poverty variables of interest
- Two map layers from the Pittsburgh City Planning Department in state plane coordinates for Parks and Neighborhoods
- A data table from City Planning defining each city neighborhood in terms of the census tracts that make up neighborhoods

You will use this data to study youth pedestrian injuries in Pittsburgh. Along the way you will use many GIS tasks and functions: extract by attribute value, clip, select, and extract features by location, edit polygons, append map layers, set data frame and map layer projections, and dissolve polygons.

Your first step is to select and extract a boundary map layer with the single polygon consisting of Pittsburgh's boundary. It serves as a "cookie cutter" for extracting Pittsburgh streets, water polygons, and census tracts from the TIGER/Line county maps. Carrying out extractions raises some interesting issues and problems. You will need to clip river polygons at the boundary of Pittsburgh to give them the same extent as the rest of Pittsburgh, otherwise they extend too far beyond Pittsburgh's boundaries. When you use the clip function in ArcToolbox, you will create new river polygon lines coinciding with Pittsburgh's boundaries. Unfortunately, some portions of the river polygons are on Pittsburgh's boundary, and Pittsburgh only extends out to the centers of the rivers. In these cases, you will edit the rivers to give them back their full width after having clipped them. While brief, this work will give you a taste of editing and creating features.

To give you practice appending map layers to make a single output map layer, we have supposed that the task of address matching the residences of injury victims was carried out by two individuals, Smith and Jones. This will break up the intense work of interactively rematching unmatched addresses and doing other work to prepare the injury point layer. So you will have to append Smith's and Jones's layers.

The next task is to start accommodating the various projection and coordinate systems of the input map layers—we have a mixture of latitude–longitude geographic and state plane rectilinear coordinates. As done in tutorial 4, you will create projection files for the city planning map layers, and you will assign a projection to the data frame for your map document. Then all layers will overlay as part of the same system.

Lastly, you will dissolve TIGER/Line census tracts to create a new version of Pittsburgh's neighborhood map layer, so your data remains TIGER-based. The version of neighborhoods obtained from City Planning was derived from tract boundaries that a City Planning GIS analyst had edited to align them with physical features in aerial photographs. When overlaying the original TIGER tracts and the City Planning neighborhoods, the result is "sliver polygons," or very narrow polygons between slightly different boundaries. So to eliminate slivers, you will replace the City Planning neighborhood layer with a new one that you create.

The analyses of this tutorial use two spatial analysis functions: intersection and buffers. You will use intersection as the basis for aggregation of point and polygon data to neighborhood polygons. You will use multiple-ring buffers to study injury rates as a function of distance from park polygons. Not much more needs to be said about these GIS analyses in this introduction, but rest assured that the work you will do is a powerful demonstration of some of the unique capabilities of GIS.

The \GistutorialHealth\PedestrianInjuries folder has several shapefiles and a data table that we downloaded from the ESRI Census 2000 TIGER/Line Data Web site (*www.esri.com /data/download/census2000_tigerline/index.html*) for Allegheny County, Pennsylvania:

  + tgr42003ccd00.shp—polygons for cities, boroughs, towns, and townships.
  + tgr42003lkA.shp—lines for street centerlines.
  + tgr42003trt00.shp—polygons for Census 2000 tracts.
  + tgr42003wat.shp—polygons for water bodies or rivers.

Also available are two point shapefiles that Smith and Jones address matched from the injury data table obtained from the pediatric hospital. The data is completely address matched with resulting points edited and moved to centers of street segments to protect privacy. These map layers are

  + InjuriesSmith.shp—half of the address matched injury points; and
  + InjuriesJones.shp—other half of the address matched injury points.

Also in the \GistutorialHealth\PedestrianInjuries folder is the data table PopPov.dbf, which we prepared from SF3 data downloaded from the Census Bureau Web site (*factfinder. census.gov/servlet/DTGeoSearchByListServlet?ds_name=DEC_2000_SF3_U&_lang=en&_ ts=154390283359*). The following attributes are in this table:

  + STFID—census tract identifier.
  + POP—total population.
  + POP5TO17—population 5 to 17 years old.
  + PCINC—per capita income.
  + POVTOT—total population below the poverty line.
  + POV5TO17—population 5 to 17 years old below the poverty line.
  + FPOVTOT = POVTOT/POP—fraction of population below the poverty line.
  + FPOV5TO17 = POV5TO17/POP5TO17—fraction of population 5 to 17 years old below the poverty line.

Finally, map layers and a data table from Pittsburgh's City Planning Department in the \GistutorialHealth\PAGIS folder include the following:

- BlockCentroids.shp—census block centroids made from census block polygons in Pittsburgh.
- Neighborhoods.shp—polygons for Pittsburgh neighborhoods, each made up of one or more census tracts.
- ParksPlaygrounds.shp—polygons for Pittsburgh parks that have playgrounds, playing fields, or other facilities for youth activities.
- tractnbd.dbf—list of every census tract identification number (STFID) and the neighborhood name to which it belongs.

Prepare study region

The first set of tasks concerns extracting Pittsburgh shapefiles from the larger Allegheny County shapefiles downloaded from the ESRI Web site. You start by extracting a boundary for Pittsburgh that you will use as a "cookie cutter" for extracting Pittsburgh shapefiles.

Extract Pittsburgh.shp

1 Start ArcMap with a new empty map.

2 Click File, Save. Name the map **Tutorial7.mxd** and save it to your **\GistutorialHealth** folder.

3 Add all of the shapefiles and tables from the **\GistutorialHealth\PedestrianInjuries** folder to the map.

4 Click the Display tab at the bottom of the table of contents, and turn off all the layers except tgr42003ccd00.shp.

5 Right-click tgr42003ccd00.shp in the table of contents and click Open Attribute Table.

6 In the resulting table, scroll down and locate the row with an **FID** value of 88 and a name value of Pittsburgh, select this record by clicking the gray row selector button at the left end of the row, then close the table.

That action results in the Pittsburgh polygon being selected.

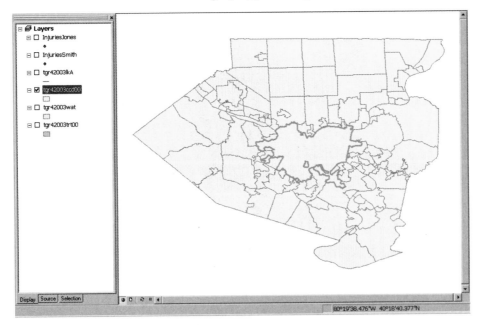

7   In the table of contents, right-click tgr42003ccd00.shp, click Data, and Export Data.

8   In the Export Data dialog box, name the output shapefile **Pittsburgh.shp** and save it in your **\GistutorialHealth\PedestrianInjuries** folder. After defining the name and location for the output, click OK and Yes to add it to your map.

9   In the table of contents, right-click tgr42003ccd00.shp and click Remove.

Pittsburgh.shp is the only layer currently displayed in your map. In upcoming steps you will use this layer to clip the water features that reside within Pittsburgh.

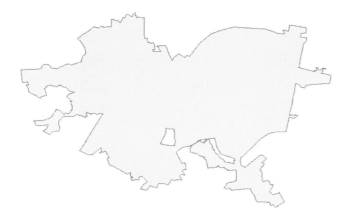

Clip water polygons

Next, you will clip the water polygons using the Pittsburgh polygon. The polygons for Pittsburgh's three major rivers extend beyond Pittsburgh's boundary, so the Clip tool will truncate those polygons at Pittsburgh's boundary.

1   If it is not already selected, click the Display tab at the bottom of the table of contents, and turn on the tgr42003wat layer. Click, hold, and drag the tgr42003wat layer just above Pittsburgh so that the rivers and other water polygons overlay the Pittsburgh boundary polygon.

2   Click the ArcToolbox icon ![icon] on the Standard toolbar.

3   In ArcToolbox, expand the Analysis Tools toolbox, then expand the Extract toolset. Inside the Extract toolset, double-click the Clip tool.

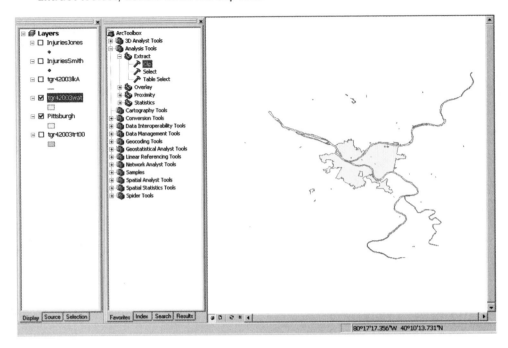

4   In the Clip dialog box, choose tgr42003wat from the Input Features drop-down list, then choose Pittsburgh from the Clip Features list. Name the Output Feature Class **Rivers.shp** and save it to your **\GistutorialHealth\PedestrianInjuries** folder. After these settings are made, click OK, and close when the Clip tool has finished processing.

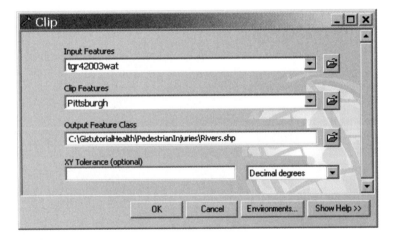

5   Close ArcToolbox.

6   Zoom to the Pittsburgh layer.

7   Click View, Bookmarks, Create, name the bookmark **Pittsburgh**, and click OK.

Edit the rivers features

The Clip tool did a nice job producing the rivers map layer, except for one problem: in places where a river is on the boundary of Pittsburgh, the boundary goes through the center of the river. In such locations, the river has half its width clipped off. You can easily remedy this problem by editing River.shp using the heads-up digitizing in ArcMap. While digitizing, you will use tgr42003wat.shp as a guide and move vertices (points) on Rivers.shp to match those of the former layer.

1   **Symbolize Pittsburgh.shp with a hollow fill and an outline width of 1.5.**

2   **Symbolize Rivers.shp with a light blue fill color.**

3   **Symbolize tgr42003wat.shp with a light orange fill color (or any color other than blue).**

4   **Use the Zoom In tool and zoom to the river layer where it intersects the western boundary of Pittsburgh.**

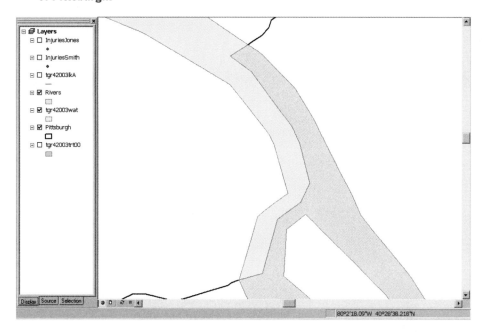

5   **If necessary, open the Editor toolbar by clicking the Editor toolbar button on the Standard toolbar.**

6   **On the Editor toolbar, click the Editor drop-down arrow and choose Start Editing. If necessary, click OK to edit the shapefiles within the \GistutorialHealth\PedestrianInjuries folder.**

7   **From the Editor menu, click Snapping.**

8   **In the upper portion of the Snapping Environment, check the Vertex box and the Edge box for the tgr42003wat layer, and close the Snapping Environment window.**

9   **On the Editor toolbar, click the Task drop-down arrow and choose Modify Feature.**

10 On the Editor toolbar, click the Target drop-down arrow and choose Rivers.

11 On the Editor toolbar, click the Edit tool ▶ and double-click anywhere on the Rivers layer in the map display.

Now you can see all of the vertices making up the rivers polygon. Next, you will edit these vertices to align them with their bounding features in tgr42003wat.shp.

12 Move your cursor over the leftmost vertex of Rivers.shp, and when the cursor icon changes to the vertex selection icon ⬥, click, hold, and drag the vertex parallel to the existing rivers line segment and drop on top of the tgr42003wat.shp boundary as shown below.

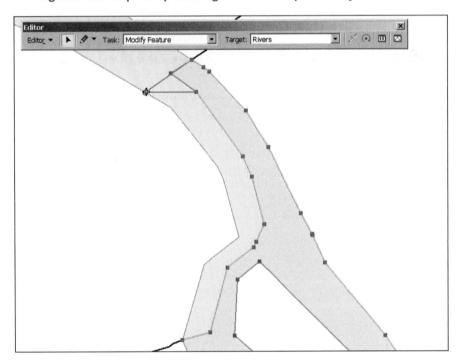

13 Continue to move the vertices in Rivers.shp so that they are coincident with the outer boundary of tgr42003wat.shp that is just outside of and following along the contour of the Pittsburgh boundary.

Hints:

+ If you run into any problems and want to start over, click the Editor button on the Edit toolbar, click Stop Editing, and do not save changes. Then start over.
+ Be sure to allow time for the vertex selection icon to appear before you try to move a vertex.
+ If a layer other than Rivers.shp gets its vertices activated, click a white area outside of Pittsburgh and then click the blue fill area of Rivers.shp to reactivate its vertices.
+ If you want to add a new vertex to Rivers.shp, right-click the Rivers.shp boundary where you'd like to add the vertex and click Insert Vertex.

14 **When you have finished editing this portion of Rivers.shp, click the Editor drop-down arrow and choose Stop Editing. Click Yes to save your edits.**

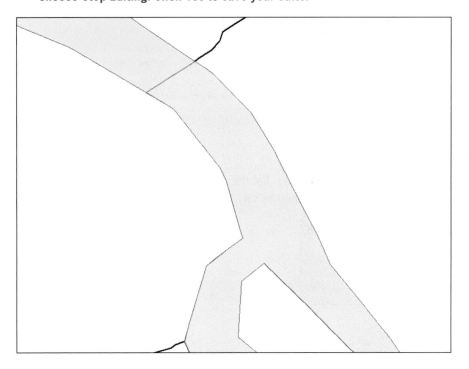

15 **Use your Pittsburgh bookmark to zoom out to see all of Pittsburgh.**

YOUR TURN

Rivers.shp has two more polygons to edit, one on the northern side of Pittsburgh and the other on the southern side. Time permitting, edit both. If time is limited, edit just one of them. Make sure that Modify Feature is the task selected on the Editor toolbar. When finished, save your edits and stop editing.

Extract streets and tracts for Pittsburgh

You should never clip street centerline segments because that would lead to location errors in address matching. If a street segment were half in Pittsburgh and half outside, the resulting street segment clipped to be inside of Pittsburgh (and half as long as the original), would still have its original attribute record and street number range. Address matching for the clipped street segment would place points for the entire range of original street numbers all within Pittsburgh, including the half of the segment actually outside of Pittsburgh. Thus, in extracting Pittsburgh streets, you will include all street segments with their original lengths that intersect with or are within Pittsburgh's boundary.

1   Turn the tgr42003lkA layer on in your map.

2   From the Selection menu, click Select By Location. Set the options in the Select By Location dialog box so that they match those in the graphic below.

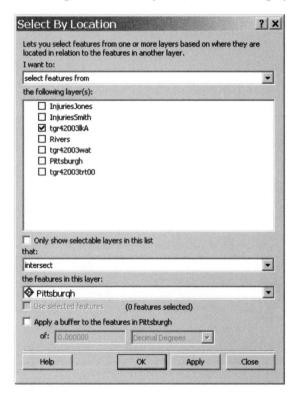

3   Click Apply and then Close.

4   In the table of contents, right-click tgr42003lkA.shp, click Data, Export Data, name the output shapefile **Streets.shp**, and save it to your **\GistutorialHealth\PedestrianInjuries** folder.

5   Click OK and Yes.

6   Turn the tgr42003lkA layer off in your map, and symbolize Streets with a light gray color.

7   **Move the Pittsburgh layer to the top of the table of contents.**

Notice that some street segments extend outside of Pittsburgh's boundary, as anticipated.

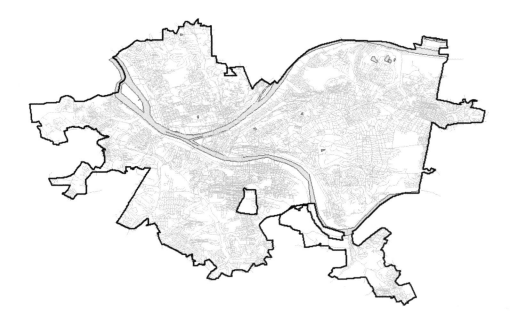

YOUR TURN

Using a similar procedure to that described in the previous steps, extract the census tracts that are within Pittsburgh. In this case, though, select the features from tgr42003trt00.shp, and in the Select By Location query, use the "Have their centroid in" function instead of "Intersect." (If you were to use Intersect, you'd also select tracts just outside of and touching Pittsburgh, which you don't want in this case.) Name the output shapefile **Tracts** and save it within your \GistutorialHealth\PedestrianInjuries folder.

Join tracts and the census data table

The Tracts shapefile, as downloaded, has no census data attached to it. We downloaded and prepared a table of desirable SF3 variables, PopPov.dbf, which you will now join to Tracts.shp.

1 **In the table of contents, right-click Tracts, click Joins and Relates, and click Join.**

2 **Set the options in the Join Data dialog box so that they match the settings shown in the graphic below.**

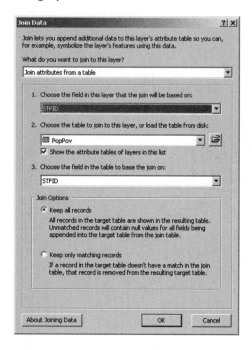

3 **Click OK.**

4 **Right-click Tracts in the table of contents and click Open Attribute Table.**

5 **Scroll to the right in the table to confirm that the attributes from the PopPov table were joined to the Tracts.**

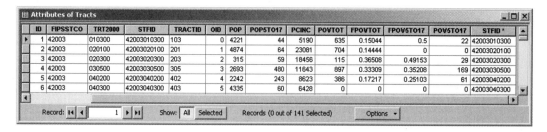

6 **Close Attributes of Tracts.**

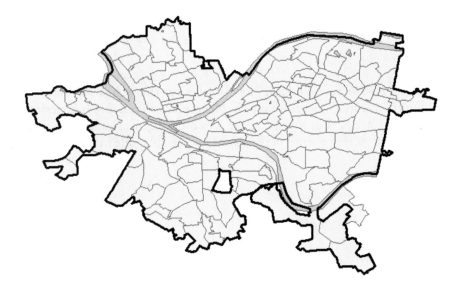

Append injury shapefiles

Next you will append the shapefile address matched by Smith to the one address matched by Jones. For two shapefiles to be appended, they must be of the same vector data type (point, line, or polygon) and have identical attribute names and field types in their feature attribute tables. This is the case for the two injury shapefiles.

1   **Click the ArcToolbox icon** 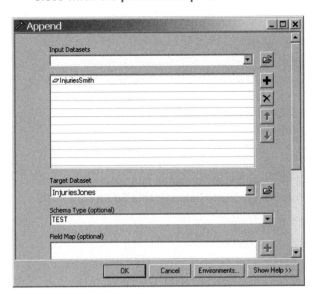 **on the Standard toolbar.**

2   **In the resulting ArcToolbox panel, expand the Data Management Tools toolbox, then the General toolset. In the General toolset, double-click the Append tool.**

3   **In the Append dialog box, click the Input Datasets drop-down arrow and choose InjuriesSmith.**

4   **From the Target Dataset list in the Append dialog box, choose InjuriesJones. Click OK, then click Close when the process completes.**

5   Close ArcToolbox.

6   Open Attributes of InjuriesJones.

Originally, InjuriesJones only had 48 rows of data. Now you can see that it has 94 rows, because you appended Smith's records (and points) to it. Next, you will rename InjuriesJones as InjuryResidences using ArcCatalog. But first you have to remove InjuriesJones from your current ArcMap session so that you have write permissions for the shapefile in ArcCatalog.

7   Close Attributes of InjuriesJones.

Clean up your map and rename a shapefile

1   Right-click InjuriesJones and click Remove, do the same for InjuriesSmith, tgr42003lkA, tgr4003wat, and tgr42003trt00 (the latter four are no longer needed).

2   Start ArcCatalog.

3   In the catalog tree, navigate to your **\GistutorialHealth\PedestrianInjuries** folder.

4   Right-click InjuriesJones in the catalog tree, click Rename, and type InjuryResidences.

5   Close ArcCatalog.

6   In ArcMap, click the Add Data button [✛] and add InjuryResidences to the map.

7   Turn on all the layers in your map except Tracts and Streets.

8   Symbolize InjuryResidences with a Circle 2 point symbol set to a Size value of 7 and a red color.

Set the projection for the data and map layers

The next set of steps assigns a state plane projection to the Layers data frame in your current map and then builds projection files for Neighborhoods.shp and ParksPlaygrounds.shp. As obtained from the Pittsburgh City Planning Department, these map layers are in state plane coordinates, but they don't currently have their projection information stored in a projection file; whereas the TIGER/Line maps already in your map, which are stored in geographic (latitude–longitude) coordinates, already have projection files, meaning that they will project on-the-fly to match the data frame's assigned projection and coordinate system.

1   In the table of contents, right-click Layers, click Properties, click the Coordinate System tab.

2   In the Select a coordinate system box, navigate to **Predefined\Projected Coordinate Systems \State Plane\NAD 1983 (Feet)** and click **NAD 1983 State Plane Pennsylvania South FIPS 3702 (Feet)**.

3   Click Apply and OK.

The data frame now has the proper state projection for Pittsburgh. Even though the TIGER/Line map layers are in geographic coordinates, ArcMap automatically projects them to state plane.

4   Zoom to the Tracts layer, and create a new bookmark named **Pittsburgh**. (Doing this will replace the existing Pittsburgh bookmark.)

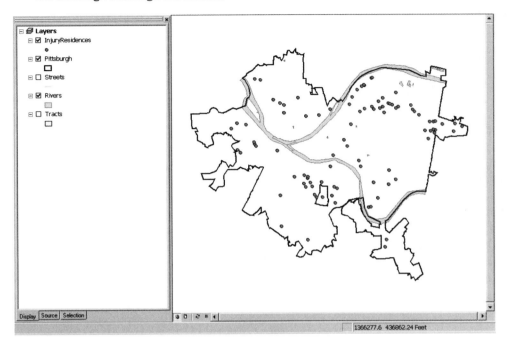

5   Start ArcCatalog.

6   In the catalog tree, navigate to the **\GistutorialHealth\PAGIS** folder.

7   Right-click **Neighborhoods.shp** and click Properties.

8   In the Shapefile Properties window, click the XY Coordinate System tab.

9   Click the Select button, navigate to **Projected Coordinate Systems\State Plane\NAD 1983 (Feet)**, and double-click **NAD 1983 StatePlane Pennsylvania South FIPS 3702 (Feet).prj**.

10 Click Apply and OK.

YOUR TURN

Use the same procedure to assign the state plane projection to ParksPlaygrounds.shp. Close ArcCatalog when finished.

Add City Planning (PAGIS) map layers

Now you will add two layers from Pittsburgh's City Planning Department: Neighborhoods.shp and ParksPlaygrounds.shp.

1   **Click the Add Data button** 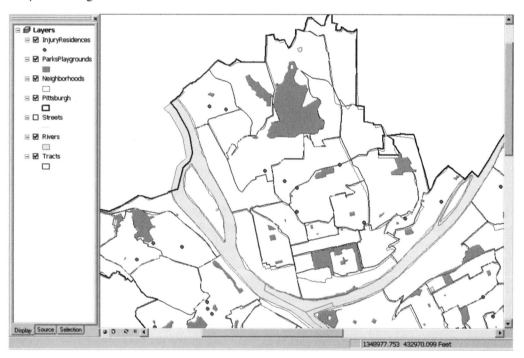**, navigate to the \GistutorialHealth\PAGIS folder, and add Neighborhoods.shp and ParksPlaygrounds.shp to the map document.**

2   **Symbolize the Neighborhoods layer with a hollow fill color and blue outline. Symbolize the ParksPlaygrounds layer with a medium green fill color. Symbolize Tracts with a hollow fill.**

3   **Turn on Tracts in your map, zoom to the northern portion of Pittsburgh above the rivers and compare the Tracts polygons with those of Neighborhoods.**

While Neighborhoods and Tracts should be coterminous, you can see that the tracts used to build neighborhoods were slightly different than the TIGER/Line tracts in your map document. The boundaries do not match perfectly so that the overlay of the two polygon layers creates small sliver polygons where there should be none. To remedy this problem, you will simply rebuild the neighborhood polygons using the tractnbd.dbf file supplied by City Planning.

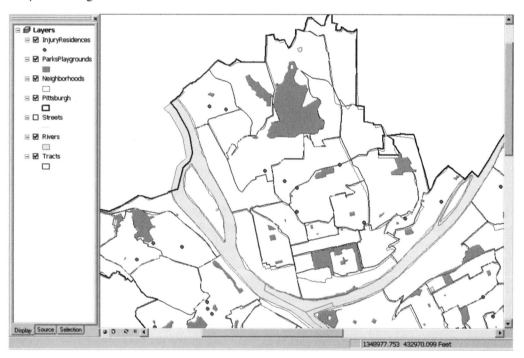

Dissolve tracts to build the neighborhoods map layer

In these steps you will use the dissolve function of ArcToolbox with the inputs of the TIGER/Line Tracts shapefile you extracted and the tractnbd.dbf table that lists each tract of a neighborhood. The dissolve function removes boundaries between adjacent polygons that have the same value for a specified value of a specified attribute.

1   Click the Add Data button 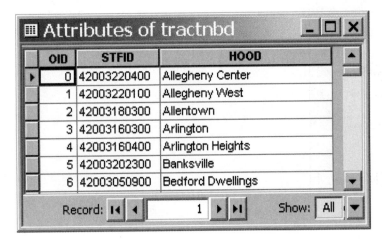, navigate to the **\GistutorialHealth\PAGIS** folder, and add **tractnbd.dbf** to the map document.

2   At the bottom of the table of contents, click the Source tab, right-click tractnbd, and click Open.

You can see that this file has the needed information to dissolve tracts into neighborhoods. STFID is the tract identifier and HOOD is the neighborhood name.

OID	STFID	HOOD
0	42003220400	Allegheny Center
1	42003220100	Allegheny West
2	42003180300	Allentown
3	42003160300	Arlington
4	42003160400	Arlington Heights
5	42003202300	Banksville
6	42003050900	Bedford Dwellings

Record: 1   Show: All

3   Close the attribute table and click the Display tab at the bottom of the table of contents.

Next, you have to join the tractnbd table to the Tracts.shp feature attribute table. Then the dissolve function will have inputs ready in the desired form.

4   In the table of contents, right-click Tracts, click Joins and Relates, click Join, and make
    selections as seen below in the Join Data dialog box.

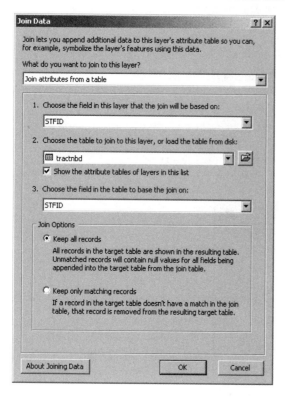

5   Click OK then Yes.

6   Click the ArcToolbox button on the Standard toolbar.

7   Navigate to and expand the Data Management Tools toolbox, then expand the Generalization
    toolset and double-click the Dissolve tool.

8   In the Dissolve dialog box, click the Input Features drop-down arrow and choose Tracts. Name
    the output feature class **NeighTracts.shp** and save it in your **\GistutorialHealth\PedestrianInjuries**
    folder. In the Dissolve_Field(s) panel, scroll to the bottom of the list of fields, then check
    tractnbd.HOOD.

9   Click OK. Click Close when the dissolve is completed.

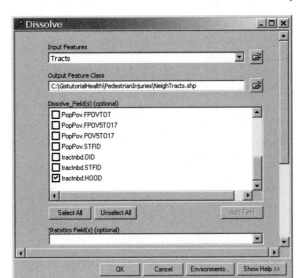

10 Close the ArcToolbox.

11 From the table of contents, remove Neighborhoods and symbolize the new NeighTracts layer with a hollow fill and blue outline.

12 Use your Pittsburgh bookmark to zoom out to see all of Pittsburgh.

Now you can see that the tracts and the new neighborhoods are coterminous. In neighborhoods made up of more than one census tract, you can see the interior black lines of Tracts that were dissolved in making the new neighborhood layer.

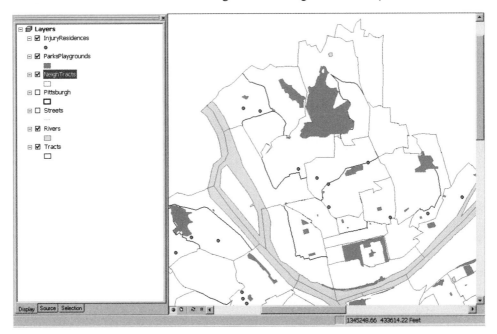

Investigate the correlation of poverty and injuries

The objective of this section is to aggregate poverty and injury data to the neighborhood level, produce a map with display of those variables at the neighborhood level, and produce a correlation coefficient for the relationship between the two variables. Aggregation of each variable requires two steps: (1) intersect NeighTracts.shp with InjuryResidences.shp or Tracts.shp to assign neighborhood identifiers to injury points or tract polygons, and (2) count injuries by neighborhood identifier and sum a poverty variable by neighborhood. This results in two aggregate datasets by neighborhood, which you will join to produce the final dataset for plotting and analysis.

Intersect map layers

First you will intersect NeighTracts polygons and InjuryResidences points to create a new point shapefile with NeighTracts data attached to each point.

1   Turn off ParkPlaygrounds, Streets (should already be off), and Tracts, and turn all other layers on.

2   Open ArcToolbox, expand the Analysis Tools toolbox and the Overlay toolset, then double-click Intersect.

3   In the Intersect dialog box, click the Input Features drop-down list and choose NeighTracts, then repeat the process and choose InjuryResidences. Name the Output Feature Class **NeighTract_Injury.shp** and save it in your **\GistutorialHealth\PedestrianInjuries** folder. Finally, scroll to the bottom of the Intersect dialog box, click the Output Type drop-down arrow, and choose POINT.

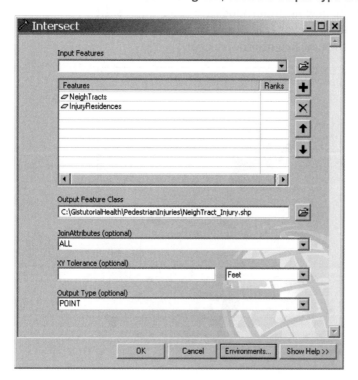

4   **Click OK and Close.**

5   **Right-click NeighTract_Injury and click Open Attribute Table.**

6   **Examine the table to see that every injury record now has its neighborhood name as a result of the intersection and then close the table.**

7   **Close the attribute table.**

TURN

YOUR

Use similar steps to intersect NeighTracts.shp and Tracts.shp. Choose Output Type=INPUT and name the output file NeighTracts_Intersect.shp. Examine the resulting intersected shapefile to see that each of the 140 tracts in Pittsburgh has its neighborhood name. You will notice that there are 141 records in the attribute table and one (FIDO) has no data. This is because it is a polygon just outside the city of Pittsburgh's boundary and can be ignored. When finished, close the attribute table and ArcToolbox.

TURN AGAIN

YOUR

The Intersect function does not include tables joined to the input layers in the resulting output layer. Hence, you need to join PopPov.dbf to the attribute table of NeighTracts_Intersect.shp using Tracts_STF and STFID as the Join columns.

Aggregate records

Here you will use the InjuryResidences point shapefile that you just created to count the number of injuries in each neighborhood.

1   **Right-click NeighTract_Injury, click Open Attribute Table, right-click the field name tractnbd_H, then choose Summarize.**

2   **In the resulting Summarize dialog box, name the output table CountInjuries.dbf and save it in your \GistutorialHealth\PedestrianInjuries folder.**

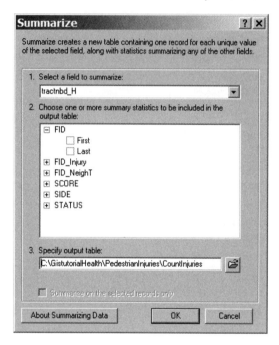

3   **Click OK and Yes.**

4   **Close the attribute table.**

5   **Click the Source tab at the bottom of the table of contents.**

6   **Right-click CountInjuries.dbf and click Open. Examine this table to see that it has the number of injuries per neighborhood.**

7   **Close the table and click the Display tab at the bottom of the table of contents.**

YOUR TURN

Sum the NeighTracts_Intersect.tractnbd_H field in the NeighTracts_Intersect layer to produce a table called SumPovPop.dbf that has the number of youth ages 5 to 17 that live in poverty per neighborhood. See the following Summarize window for selections needed.

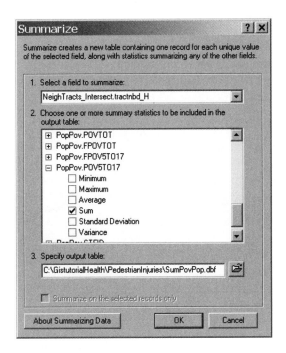

Resultant table of population ages 5 to 17 in poverty for each neighborhood.

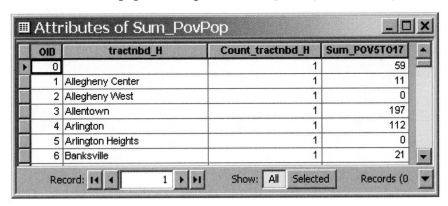

Join tables

Next, you will join the number of injuries in each neighborhood (CountInjuries) to the summary table you created in the previous Your turn that shows the poverty population ages 5 to 17 in neighborhoods, and then join this to the shapefile of neighborhoods and census tracts.

1   **In the table of contents, click the Source tab, right-click SumPovPop.dbf, click Joins and Relates, and click Join.**

2   **In the resulting Join Data dialog box, make selections as shown and click OK.**

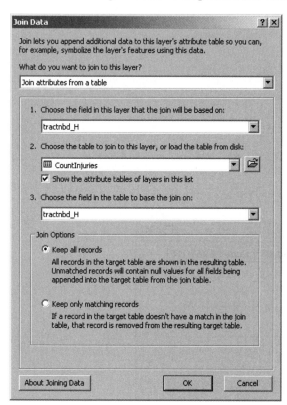

3   **Right-click SumPovPop, click Open, and see that you now have a record for each neighborhood with neighborhood-level data for injuries and youth poverty population.**

The null values indicated in the table are expected: they are for neighborhoods that do not have injuries.

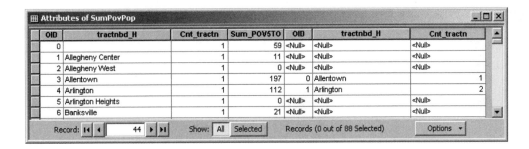

OID	tractnbd_H	Cnt_tractn	Sum_POV5TO	OID	tractnbd_H	Cnt_tractn
0		1	59	<Null>	<Null>	<Null>
1	Allegheny Center	1	11	<Null>	<Null>	<Null>
2	Allegheny West	1	0	<Null>	<Null>	<Null>
3	Allentown	1	197	0	Allentown	1
4	Arlington	1	112	1	Arlington	2
5	Arlington Heights	1	0	<Null>	<Null>	<Null>
6	Banksville	1	21	<Null>	<Null>	<Null>

Record: ◄◄ ◄ 44 ► ►◄   Show: All Selected   Records (0 out of 88 Selected)   Options ▾

4   **Close the Attributes of SumPovPop table.**

5   **Remove the NeighTract_Injury and NeighTracts_Intersect layers from the table of contents.**

6   **Right-click NeighTracts, click Joins and Relates, then Join, and make selections as shown below, then click OK.**

Note: The SumPovPop table shows up as SumPovPop_CountInjuries in the drop-down list for item 2 below. Make that selection. In item 3, choose the first of the two tractnbd_H fields.

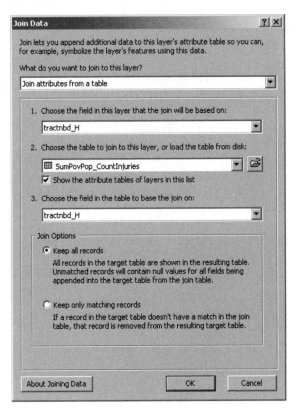

The resultant table contains records for each neighborhood/tract with a count of injuries and poverty population within each.

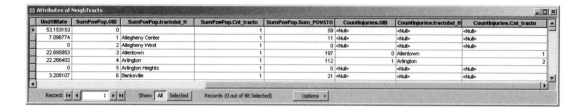

7 Close the Attributes of NeighTracts table.

Symbolize map layers

Within this set of steps, you will symbolize the layers to show by neighborhood the number of children living in poverty compared to the injury locations.

1 **Click the Display tab at the bottom of the table of contents.**

2 **Right-click NeighTracts, click Properties, then click the Symbology tab.**

3 **In the Show panel, click Quantities, Graduated colors. From the Value drop-down list, choose Sum_POV5T017.**

4 **Click the Classify button. In the Classification dialog box, choose Quantile from the Method drop-down list, then click OK.**

5 **In the Symbol list shown on the Symbology tab, double-click the symbol associated with the 0–22 range, and change its color to a bright blue color (e.g., Yogo Blue), and click OK.**

6 **Continue down the list of symbols by making the following symbol color sections for each value range: 23-66, Sugilite Sky; 67-137, Arctic White; 138-225, Mango; and 226-838, Seville Orange. Once the colors are all set for all the symbols, click OK to close the Layer Properties.**

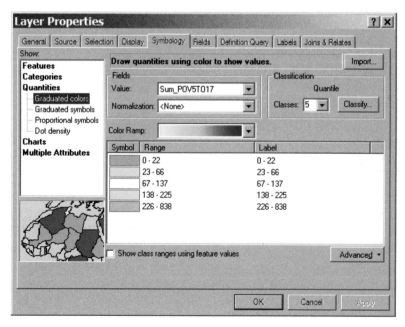

Now you can see the neighborhoods that have children living in poverty. The top 40 percent of neighborhoods, seen in shades of orange, clearly have more injuries than the lowest 40 percent of neighborhoods, seen in shades of blue. Next you will start to quantify this relationship.

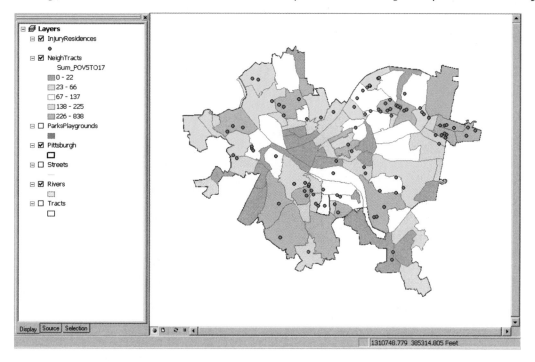

Count injuries by top and bottom 40 percent quantiles

Now that you have map layers showing locations of injury and poverty, it is easy to calculate if neighborhoods with high poverty are those where injuries are occurring.

1   Click the Selection menu and click Select by Attributes.

2   In the Select By Attributes window, choose NeighTracts from the Layer drop-down list, double-click "Sum_PovPop.Sum_POV5TO" in the list of fields, click the >= button, and type **138** into the lower panel after the >= sign.

Those actions build an attribute query to select all neighborhoods in the top 40 percent of youth population living in poverty.

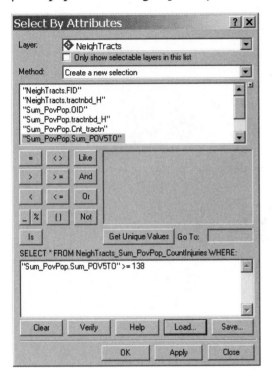

3   Click OK.

The resultant map shows neighborhoods with high poverty selected.

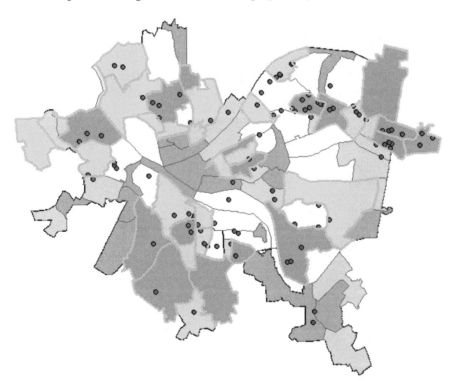

4   Click the Selection menu, click Select By Location. Within the Select By Location dialog box, make the settings shown below.

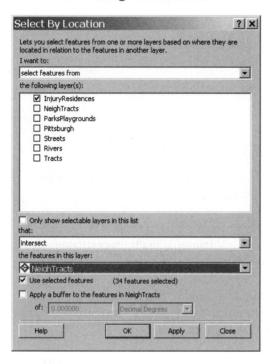

5   Click Apply and Close.

6   Open the Attributes of InjuryResidences table.

From the resulting selection statistics of InjuryResidences, you will find that 61 of 94 injuries (66 percent) fall into the top 40 percent of neighborhoods by youth population living in poverty. That's a good indication that poverty is a factor in serious youth pedestrian injuries.

7   If necessary, close any open attribute tables.

8   Click the Selection menu and click Clear Selected Features.

9   Save the project as **C:\GistutorialHealth\Tutorial7.mxd**.

YOUR TURN

Determine the number of injuries in the lowest 40 percent of neighborhoods by youth poverty population. Hint: The attribute selection criterion needed is "Sum_PovPop.Sum_POV5TO" <= 67 and the result is only 13 out of 94 injuries (14 percent) are in the lowest youth poverty population neighborhoods. Clear the selection.

If you were to calculate the correlation coefficient for Sum_POV5TO (the youth population in poverty by neighborhood) and count_tractnbd_H (number of injuries per neighborhood), you would find a rather high correlation of 0.581 between these variables.

Investigate injuries near parks

Your last task in this tutorial is to conduct a proximity analysis of parks and serious youth pedestrian injuries. You will use ArcToolbox to construct 600- and 1,200-foot buffers around parks and then analyze injury rates per 10,000 youths in the 0- to 600-foot and 600- to 1,200-foot rings around parks. We expect injury rates to be higher for youths living in the 600- to 1,200-foot ring.

Build multiple-ring buffers

1   **Turn off NeighTracts, Streets, and Tracts layers in your map, and turn on all other layers.**

2   **If necessary, open ArcToolbox. In ArcToolbox, navigate to the Analysis Tools toolbox, then the Proximity toolset, and double-click the Multiple Ring Buffer tool.**

3   **In the Multiple Ring Buffer dialog box, choose ParksPlaygrounds from the Input Features list, name the output features ParksBuffers, and save it in your \GistutorialHealth\PedestrianInjuries folder. Type 0.5 in the Distances box and click the plus (+) button.**

That enters the distance of the first buffer and amounts to a "trick." You need the ring from 0 to 600 feet, but the multiple-ring buffer cannot use the value 0 as an input. Instead, you have to use a small value, near zero, for which we had you use 0.5 foot.

4   **Type 600 in the Distances field and click the plus button, then enter a distance value of 1200.**

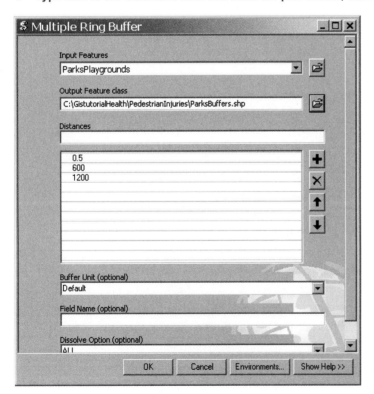

5   Click OK and Close. Close ArcToolbox.

6   Right-click ParksBuffers, click Properties, and click the Symbology tab.

7   In the Show panel, click the Quantities, then Graduated colors. From the Value drop-down list, choose Distance.

8   In the Symbol list, double-click the symbol associated with the 0.5 range value and set the symbology to a hollow fill. For the other two symbols in this list use light and medium gray colors. Once the symbology is defined, click OK.

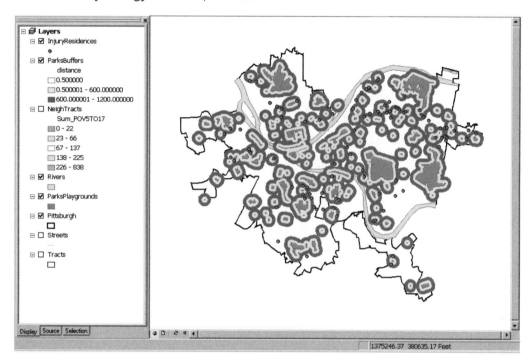

Analyze injuries and population using buffers

Here you will select injury and block centroid points within the park buffers to determine injury rates within the 600- and 1,200-foot buffers.

1   Add **BlockCentroids.shp** to your map from the **\GistutorialHealth\PAGIS** folder.

2   Symbolize the layer using a Circle 1 point symbol with a medium gray color and a size of 2.

3   Right-click ParksBuffers, click Open Attribute Table. In the table, click the gray row selector button in the second row that has a distance value of 600, and close the attribute table.

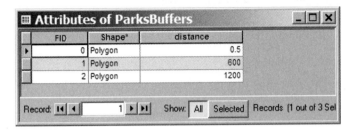

4   Click the Selection menu, click Select By Location, and match the settings shown in the following screen capture.

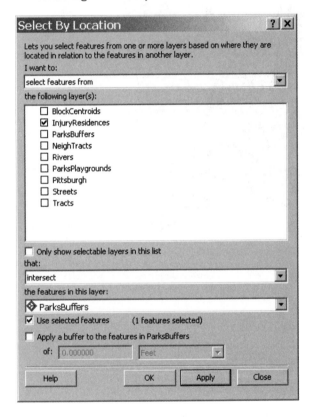

5   Click Apply and Close.

6   Right-click InjuryResidences, click Open Attribute Table and note that there are 28 injuries in the 600-foot buffer.

7   Close the attribute table.

8   Click the Selection menu, click Select By Location, and match the settings shown below.

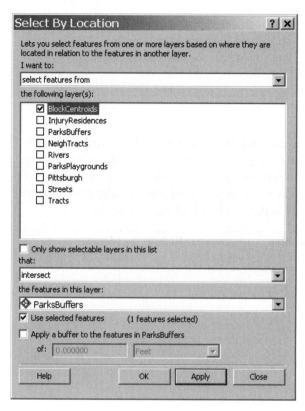

9   Click Apply and Close.

10 Right-click BlockCentroids, click Open Attribute Table, right-click the AGE_5_17 field name, click Statistics, and note that there is a sum of 15,143 youths in the 600-foot buffer.

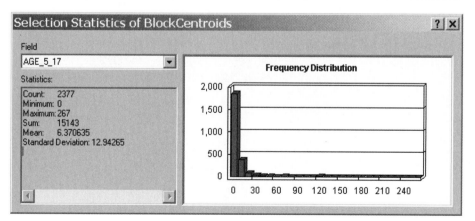

11 Close the Selection Statistics of BlockCentroids window and close the attribute table.

12 Click Selection, Clear Selected Features.

13 Save the project as **Tutorial7-2.mxd.**

YOUR TURN

Repeat the above analysis to get the number of injuries and sum of youths in the 600- to 1,200-foot buffer, with distance 1,200. You will find that there are 43 injuries and 16,947 youths in the 600- to 1,200-foot buffer ring. When finished, save your map document and close ArcMap.

The table below summarizes the results you have found. Injuries per 10,000 youths are 37 percent higher in the 600- to 1,200-foot buffer ring than in the 0- to 600-foot buffer ring, suggesting that youths living in the 600-foot buffer ring have relatively fewer serious injuries. We speculate this is because the latter youths play more in parks, which are safer environments removed from vehicular traffic. The ratio of 1.37 is derived by dividing 25.4 by 18.5.

Ring	Injuries	Youth population	Injuries per 10,000 youths	Ratio
0–600	28	15,143	18.5	1.00
600–1,200	43	16,947	25.4	1.37

Summary

You have investigated hypothesized relationships between serious youth pedestrian injuries in Pittsburgh and two explanatory variables: poverty and access to parks. We expected that injury rates would increase with poverty levels and decrease with proximity to parks. The basis of this work was a sample of 94 injuries collected over a five-year period by a pediatric hospital—a relatively small number of cases compared to the population of 90 Pittsburgh neighborhoods. For this reason and others, this study was highly exploratory.

Nevertheless, we found some evidence to support both hypotheses. A total of 66 percent of serious youth injury residences are in the top 40 percent of neighborhoods by number of youths living in poverty, whereas, only 14 percent of such injuries are in the lowest 40 percent of neighborhoods by youth poverty population. The simple correlation between the number of injuries by neighborhood and total youth living in poverty by neighborhood is nearly 0.6 (0.581). We also found that the serious injury rate per 10,000 youths is 37 percent higher in the 600- to 1,200-foot buffer ring of parks, compared to the 0- to 600-foot buffer ring. This supports the hypothesis that living near parks reduces youth pedestrian injuries.

In future work, we hope to use a larger sample of injury data, for example, one that also includes moderate injuries from all Pittsburgh hospitals. We could do better if we obtained accident location addresses, in addition to residence addresses of victims. Also, it seems relevant to start including more physical features as explanatory variables, such as nature and actual locations of play facilities.

This tutorial provided a nice recap and extension of many skills you learned in tutorials 1 through 6. If you successfully completed the tutorial, you have acquired nearly every skill needed to use GIS to study a region of interest that is not a county or a state.

The work accomplished in this tutorial illustrates the unique and powerful spatial analysis capabilities of GIS. Spatial joins are key to data aggregation—transforming individual events into aggregate measures to use in modeling. Buffers provide a way to study the impact of proximity of populations to facilities. The next tutorial takes spatial analysis to another level, asking you to spatially interpolate data—a common task facing analysts who study spatial phenomena.

Exercise assignment 7-1

Additional sensitivity analysis

Problem:

In the last task of tutorial 7, you conducted a proximity analysis of parks and serious youth pedestrian injuries using 600- and 1,200-foot buffers. In this exercise, you will rerun the buffer analysis with buffers of 1,320 feet (.25 miles) and 1,500 feet (.28 miles) and compare this with the results of the buffer analysis in the tutorial.

Start with the following:

- **C:\GistutorialHealth\PAGIS\Neighborhoods.shp**—polygon shapefile of Pittsburgh city neighborhoods with the projection added in tutorial 7.

- **C:\GistutorialHealth\PAGIS\BlockCentroids.shp**—point centroids for youth population in the city of Pittsburgh.

- **C:\GistutorialHealth\PAGIS\ParksAndPlaygrounds.shp**—polygon shapefile of parks and playgrounds in the city of Pittsburgh with the projection added in tutorial 7.

- **C:\GistutorialHealth\SolutionComponents\Chapter7\InjuryResidences.shp**—point shapefile of pedestrian injuries joined from InjurySmith.shp and InjuryJones.shp in tutorial 7.

Do additional sensitivity analysis for buffers around parks

Begin a new project called C:\GistutorialHealth\Answers\Assignment7\Assignment7-1.mxd that includes a map layout with a buffer analysis of parks and number of injuries, sum of youths, and ratio using buffers of 1,320 and 1,500 feet. Repeat the analysis that you performed in tutorial 7 using new buffers of 0–1,320 and 1,320–1,500 feet.

Add the analysis results to the table you created in tutorial 7 comparing the number of injuries to youths in the 600- and 1,200-foot buffers. Save the new table in a Word document called C:\GistutorialHealth\Answers\Assignment7\Assignment7.doc.

Export your map to a PDF file called C:\GistutorialHealth\Answers\Assignment7\Assignment7-1.pdf.

Save new shapefiles in C:\GistutorialHealth\Answers\Assignment7.

Exercise assignment 7-2

Map injuries near schools and convenience stores

Problem:

Pedestrian injuries may also occur near swimming pools, convenience stores, and other likely neighborhood kids' destinations. Children are sometimes injured near schools on weekends, holidays, or on school days when they return to play on school grounds after crossing guards have gone and school-zone lights are no longer flashing.

In this exercise you will run a buffer analysis similar to those you did for parks but this time for schools and convenience stores in the city of Pittsburgh.

Start with the following:

- **C:\GistutorialHealth\PAGIS\Neighborhoods.shp**—polygon shapefile of Pittsburgh city neighborhoods with the projection added in tutorial 7.

- **C:\GistutorialHealth\PAGIS\BlockCentroids.shp**—point centroids for youth population in the city of Pittsburgh.

- **C:\GistutorialHealth\PAGIS\Schools.shp**—point shapefile of Pittsburgh schools.

- **C:\GistutorialHealth\PAGIS\ConvenienceStores.shp**—point shapefile of convenience stores in the city of Pittsburgh.

- **C:\GistutorialHealth\SolutionComponents\Chapter7\InjuryResidences.shp**—point shapefile of pedestrian injuries joined from InjurySmith.shp and InjuryJones.shp in tutorial 7.

Do a sensitivity analysis of injuries for buffers around schools and convenience stores

Create a new project called C:\GistutorialHealth\Answers\Assignment7\Assignment7-2.mxd with a layout that includes a 600- and 1,200-foot buffer analysis around schools. Create another table in the Word document from 7-1 showing the number of injuries, sum of youth, and ratio in the 600- and 1,200-foot buffers around schools. Repeat the buffer analysis and table for convenience stores and serious pedestrian injuries.

Export the map as a JPEG file called C:\GistutorialHealth\Answers\Assignment7\Assignment7-2.jpg.

Save new shapefiles in C:\GistutorialHealth\Answers\Assignment7.

What to turn in:

If you are working in a classroom setting with an instructor, you may be required to submit the exercises you created in chapter 7. Below are the files you are required to turn in. Be sure to use a compression program such as PKZIP or WinZip to include all files as one ZIP document for review and grading. Include your name and assignment number in the ZIP document <YourNameAssignment7.zip>.

ArcMap projects

C:\GistutorialHealth\Answers\Assignment7\Assignment7-1.mxd
C:\GistutorialHealth\Answers\Assignment7\Assignment7-2.mxd

New files

C:\GistutorialHealth\Answers\Assignment7\ParksBuffer2.shp
C:\GistutorialHealth\Answers\Assignment7\SchoolsBuffer.shp
C:\GistutorialHealth\Answers\Assignment7\ConvenienceStoresBuffer.shp

Word document

C:\GistutorialHealth\Answers\Assignment7\Assignment7.doc

Exported maps

C:\GistutorialHealth\Answers\Assignment7\Assignment7-1.pdf
C:\GistutorialHealth\Answers\Assignment7\Assignment7-2.jpg

OBJECTIVES

Use spatial joins to aggregate data
Use indicator variables and spatial joins to apportion data
Build a model for automating apportionment

GIS Tutorial 8

Transform data using approximate methods

Health-care scenario

Analysis of health policy issues generally depends on area data—such as the number of infected persons per ZIP Code or the number of uninsured persons per census tract—obtained from many sources and for different types of polygon boundary layers. For mapping and modeling, it is often necessary to transform data to a common set of polygons, for example, from census tracts to health administrative territories, or from census block groups to ZIP Codes. As you will see below, it is generally reasonable to transform data from smaller areas to larger areas, but the reverse is not recommended. In some cases there will be no errors in transformation, but many cases require approximations that we hope will result in acceptable errors.

The Dartmouth Atlas of Health Care Project of the Center for the Evaluative Clinical Sciences at Dartmouth Medical School (*www.dartmouthatlas.org*) brings together researchers in diverse disciplines—including epidemiology, economics, and statistics—to describe how medical resources are distributed and used in the United States. Using very large health-care claims databases—including Medicare, Blue Cross organizations, and other sources of data—this project makes it possible to address some fundamental issues affecting the U.S. health-care system, including undesirable variations in the quality of health care across the country.

Analysts working on the Dartmouth project defined hospital service areas (local health-care markets for hospital care) and hospital referral regions (regional markets for tertiary medical care) as the appropriate geography for health-care analysis. Unfortunately, these areas are not coterminous with census area boundaries; that is, they were not constructed by aggregating census block groups or tracts. Thus, the census areas overlap research regions, and it is not possible to simply aggregate census data to the research regions. So, if analyses are to include demographic and economic data, some spatial processing is necessary to transform and, in some cases, split or apportion census data across health-service areas and health-referral regions.

A similar data transformation problem exists for analysts working for health-care organizations at the regional level. Much health-care data—such as insurance claim information, patient locations, or health complaints—is available by ZIP Code. ZIP Codes are administrative areas designed for efficient delivery of the mail. As such, they are different from census tract or other census areas, and often cross over census tract boundaries and political boundaries of towns, counties, and even states. Census 2000 Summary File 3 (SF3) data includes attributes on income, poverty, employment, educational attainment, and other variables of interest that are not available by ZIP Code or blocks. So, if SF3 variables are needed to explain variations in health-care data, they will have to be apportioned to ZIP Code areas from the smallest-sized polygons available—census block groups.

Solution approach

Three situations face the GIS analyst in transforming aggregate data spatially. Let's call the current polygons of the variable being transformed the "source polygons"; and the desired polygons after transformation the "target polygons." If the source polygons are smaller than and coterminous with the target polygons, then a simple data aggregation of source polygon variables is the solution. An example is transforming census tract data to county polygons (figure 8.1). A simple data query will sum tract data by county, and then the resultant county-level data can be joined to a county polygon map layer.

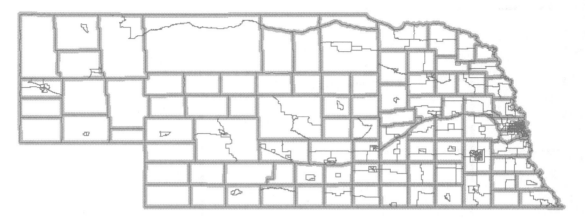

Figure 8.1   County and coterminous census tract boundaries in Nebraska.

Sources: (a) Census 2000 TIGER/Line Data; (b) ESRI Data & Maps 2005.

The second case is when the source polygons are much smaller than the target polygons but noncoterminous. The example that we use in the tutorial below is extremely safe and accurate, with over 10,000 source polygons per target polygon. Then the approach is still simple and depends on the error cancellation for accuracy. You convert the source polygons into centroid points, then perform a spatial join of the target polygons with the centroids to associate a source polygon with a single target polygon. Finally, an aggregation of centroid data by target polygon—achieved by summing the centroid data by target polygon—completes the process. In the final data, some source polygons cross target polygons, resulting in errors because each source polygon's data is only allocated to a single target polygon. This is the target polygon in which its centroids lie, where the data should be split between two or more polygons. Having a much smaller source than target polygons means that there will be many such errors per target polygon, and the errors will tend to cancel each other out. You will use this version of simple data aggregation in the first part of this tutorial.

The third approach is used when source and target polygons are comparable in size, with the source polygons at least somewhat smaller. Then cancellation of errors associated with allocating all of a source polygon's data to one target polygon does not work because there are too few source polygons per target polygon. An example is census tracts as source polygons and ZIP Codes as target polygons, where there are only four or so tracts per ZIP Code. In this case, it is necessary to split up the attribute variable of interest of a source polygon that crosses two or more target polygon boundaries and to make allocations to each target polygon.

An example is shown in figure 8.2, which displays all the census tracts within or intersected by Nebraska ZIP Code 68164. We selected tracts that cross the ZIP Code boundary so that you can see them readily. If you were to allocate census tract data to ZIP Code 68164 using census tract centroids and spatial overlay, then the ZIP Code would have none of the data from tracts 31055007309 and 31055007308, but would have all of the data from tract 31055007440 (it looks like that tract's centroid is in the ZIP Code and near its boundary). Very likely, there would be a sizable error in the resulting ZIP Code estimate of the census variable of interest.

Thus, you need an approximate means for splitting the source polygon's data. Suppose that a source polygon is split into two parts, one in target polygon A and the other in target polygon B. A simple approach is to assume that the actual split of the source polygon's

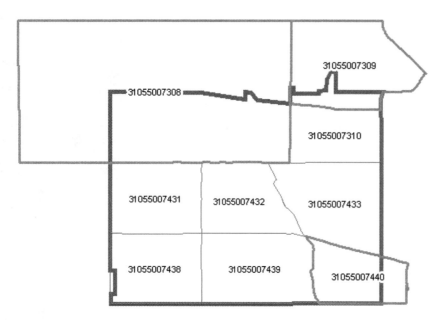

Figure 8.2 ZIP Code 68164 of Nebraska and intersecting or interior census tracts.

Sources: (a) U.S. Census Bureau; (b) Census 2000 TIGER/Line Data.

variable is proportional to its area in A and B. Then the analyst can approximately split, or apportion, the attribute to A and B using the proportions of the source's polygon in A and B as weights. Take the case of tract 31055007308: 68 percent of its area is outside ZIP Code 68164 and 32 percent is inside. If the SF3 tract variable of interest had a value of 1,000, then you would assign (apportion) $0.32 \times 1,000 = 320$ to ZIP Code 68164.

People and other entities, however, often are not distributed uniformly across areas, as is assumed for this approach, which leads to potentially sizable errors. For example, very few or no persons live in parks, lakes, or agricultural fields, all of which have area. A better approximation is to use short-form SF1 census variables, such as total population, available at the census-block level as an indicator variable for apportionment. You would assume that the SF3 variable of interest is proportional in its spatial distribution to the SF1 indicator variable.

In this case, the indicator data is joined to block centroid points and then the centroids are assigned to source and target polygons. The proportion of the source indicator variable in A and B is the basis of apportionment. The assumption here is that the attribute of interest is uniformly distributed over the indicator population of the source polygon, which is often a reasonable assumption for small locales. The attractiveness of this approach, relative to using area as the apportionment variable, is that it accounts for uninhabitable areas such as lakes, cemeteries, and so forth. You will use the block-population-based apportionment in the second part of this tutorial.

Referring back to figure 8.2, if the SF1 population variable for tract 31055007308 had a total of 8,000 with a split of 6,000 inside ZIP Code 68164 and 2,000 outside, then the apportionment fraction would be $6,000/8,000 = 0.75$ for allocating the SF3 tract data to the ZIP Code. If the SF3 tract variable of interest again had a value of 1,000, then its apportionment to the ZIP Code would be $0.75 \times 1,000 = 750$.

Aggregate block data for elderly population to health-referral regions

Census block polygons in Nebraska are not coterminous with health referral region polygons: some blocks overlap the much larger boundaries of health-referral regions. Following is an example: the selected block is split between two health-referral regions whose boundary is the dark gray line.

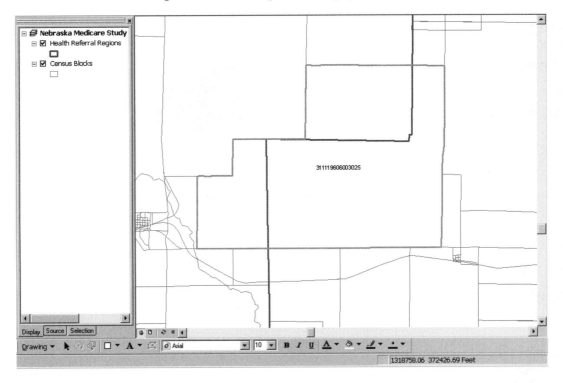

In this example, aggregating SF1 data at the block level to health-referral areas fits into the situation where the source polygons are much smaller than the target polygons but noncoterminous. So you will proceed to use simple aggregation and create block centroids from block polygons and aggregate an SF1 attribute to health-referral polygons, using a spatial join. We have already downloaded blocks for Nebraska and permanently joined the SF1 attribute of interest, AGE_65_UP, for the population aged 65 and older.

Open an existing map

1   **Launch ArcMap and open Tutorial8-1.mxd from your \GistutorialHealth folder.**

A choropleth map opens with health-referral regions in Nebraska displaying Medicare enrollees CMHS (Continuous Medicare History Sample) as 5 percent.

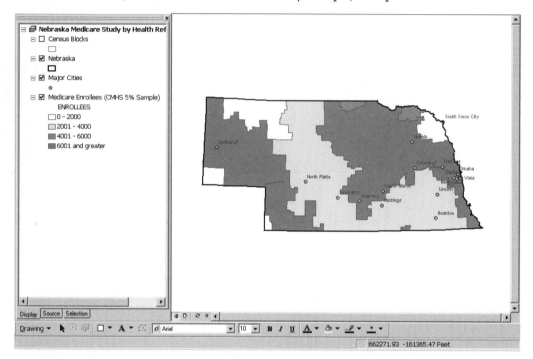

YOUR TURN

Turn on the Census Blocks layer in your map to see that there are many blocks per referral region. Then use the half-dozen bookmarks that we provided to see overlaps of blocks across referral areas. Some are small and others large. Then zoom out to the full extent and turn blocks back off.

Compute block centroid coordinates

You will use the Calculate Geometry function to calculate the X and Y centroids for each census block.

1   In the table of contents, right-click Census Blocks and click Open Attribute Table.

2   Click the Options button and Add Field.

3   In the resulting Add Field dialog box, type X in the Name field, select Double for Type, and click OK.

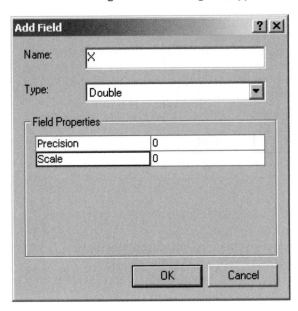

4   In the attribute table, right-click the column heading X, click Calculate Geometry, and Yes.

5   In the Calculate Geometry dialog box, click X Coordinate of Centroid from the Property drop-down list.

6   Click the radio button for "Use coordinate system of the data frame."

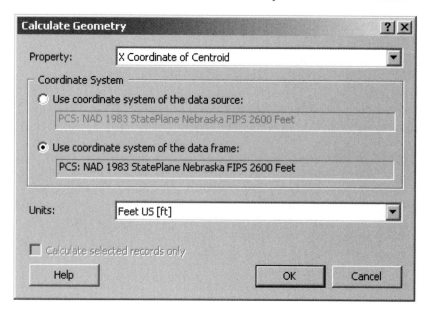

7   Click OK.

This calculation takes some time to process. Once the X field is calculated, you have completed the steps for calculating the x-coordinates of block polygon centroids.

YOUR TURN

Repeat steps 3–7 above to create the y-coordinates for the block polygon centroids. Create a new attribute called Y in the Census Blocks attribute table and use the VBA code to create the y-coordinate of a polygon centroid. When finished, close the Attributes of Census Blocks table and the Help window if open.

Here are the finished coordinates for the first few rows:

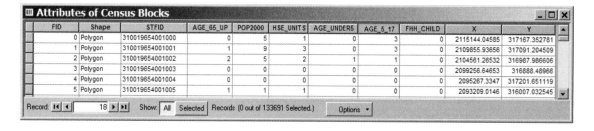

Create a block centroid shapefile

Next you will add the Census Blocks attribute table as an XY layer and then export it as a shapefile. These are necessary steps for creating the block centroid point shapefile.

1 **Click Start, My Computer, and browse to your \GistutorialHealth\Nebraska folder.**

2 **Right-click NebraskaBlocks.dbf and click Copy.**

3 **Right-click in a white area of the files panel of the Nebraska folder and click Paste. A copy of NebraskaBlocks.dbf is added to the list.**

This step is necessary for ArcMap to be able to use the blocks attribute table, which now has the x,y coordinates for centroids, as the source of an event file. ArcMap will not let you directly use the attribute table of a shapefile, hence, the copy.

4 **Close the Nebraska folder.**

5 **In ArcMap, click Tools, Add XY Data, and fill in the dialog box to match the image below. (You will need to browse to the Copy of NebraskaBlocks.dbf file.)**

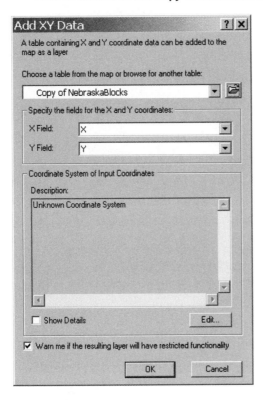

6   Click OK.

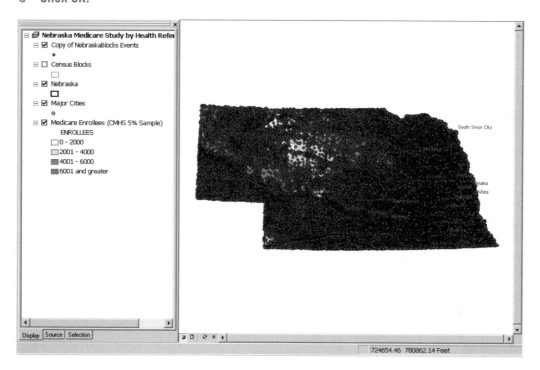

7   In the table of contents, right-click Copy of NebraskaBlocks Events and click Data and Export Data.

8   In the resulting Export Data window, name the output shapefile **BlockCentroids** and save it in your **\GistutorialHealth\Nebraska** folder, then click OK and Yes.

9   In the table of contents, right-click Copy of NebraskaBlocks Events and click Remove.

Assign block centroids a spatial reference

When you created block centroids, through the route of creating an x,y shapefile, you lost the spatial reference in the process (Nebraska state plane). Yet, the spatial join that you are about to do after this step needs accurate location information to succeed. Hence, you have to add the correct spatial reference to BlockCentroids, which you can import from NebraskaBlocks.shp.

1   Click the ArcToolbox button.

2   In ArcToolbox, navigate to the Data Management Tools toolbox, then expand the Projections and Transformations toolset.

3   Double-click the Define Projection tool.

4   From the Input Dataset or Feature Class drop-down list, choose BlockCentroids.

5   Click the Coordinate System Properties button.

6   In the Spatial Reference Properties dialog box, click the Select button.

7   In the Browse for Coordinate System dialog box, navigate to **Projected Coordinate Systems\State Plane\NAD 1983 (Feet)**, click **NAD_1983_StatePlane_Nebraska_FIPS_2600_Feet.prj**, then click Add and OK.

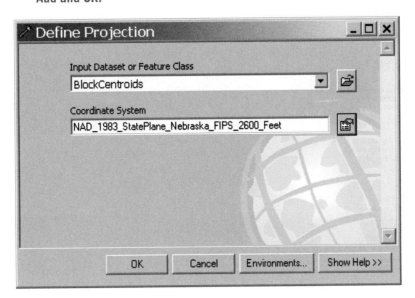

8   Click OK, then close.

Spatially join health-referral areas to block centroids

In this step, you will assign health-referral area identifiers and data to each block centroid. With this additional data, you will be able to sum the block population 65 and older to the health-referral level.

1   In the table of contents, right-click BlockCentroids, click Joins and Relates, then Join.

2   In the Join Data dialog box, make the settings match the screenshot on the following page.

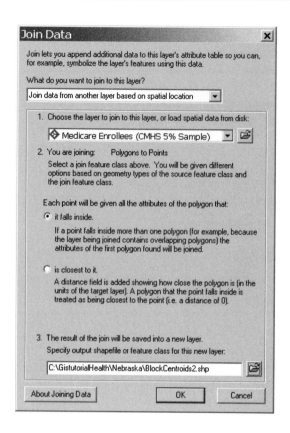

3 Click OK.

Aggregate (sum) block data to the health-referral region level

1 Open the BlockCentroids2 attribute table to see that each block has the HRR_ LABEL field.

2 Right-click the HRR_ LABEL field name and click Summarize.

3 In the Summarize dialog box, expand the AGE_65_UP field, and check Sum. Name the output table **HRRAge65Plus.dbf** and save it to your **\GistutorialHealth\Nebraska** folder.

4 Click OK then Yes to add the resultant table to the map.

5 Close the Attributes of BlockCentroids2 table.

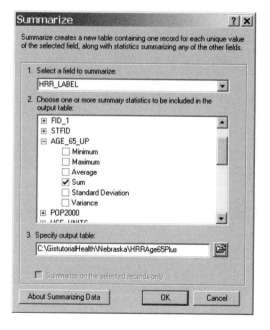

Join the new aggregate data to health-referral region

1   Remove the BlockCentroids2, BlockCentroids, and Census Blocks layers from your map.

2   Click the Add Data button 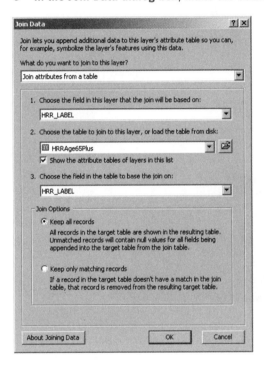 and add **NebraskaHRR.shp**.

3   If necessary, click the Display tab on the bottom of the table of contents, drag Major Cities to the top of the table of contents, then place the Nebraska layer just below it.

4   In the table of contents, right-click NebraskaHRR, click Joins and Relates, then Join.

5   In the Join Data dialog box, make the settings match the screen capture below, then click OK.

6   Right-click NebraskaHRR, then click Properties and the Symbology tab.

7   In the Symbology tab, make the classifications and settings match the screen capture on the next page, then click OK.

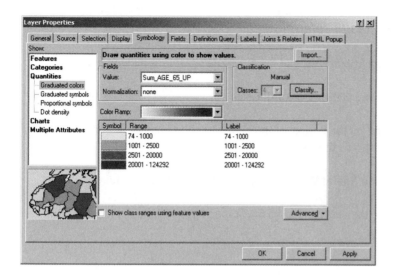

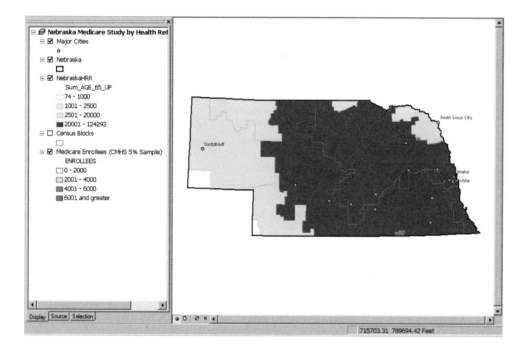

8   Save the map document as **\GistutorialHealth\Tutorial8-1.mxd** and close ArcMap.

Apportion SF3 data

In the next part of the tutorial, you will process spatial data using ArcToolbox, instead of the usual ArcMap menu selections, because you can later automate the resulting procedures by building an ArcToolbox model. You can implement any series of interactive ArcToolbox steps as a macro or model that you can run as a single step. This saves time, errors, and having to "reinvent the wheel" for a complex series of steps that you will reuse. Apportionment is an ideal candidate for an ArcToolbox model.

Below is a brief description of the shapefiles and tables in the C:\GistutorialHealth\DouglasCounty folder for input into apportionment. Included are listings of all attributes and six records for each attribute table. All shapefiles are for Douglas County, Nebraska, and have latitude–longitude coordinates. We downloaded all shapefiles and data tables from the U.S. Census Bureau and ESRI Web sites. Then we renamed files to make them more recognizable, deleted extra attributes, and renamed some attributes for clarity.

BlkGrpSF3—Table with data from the source polygons (block groups) and several SF3 attributes not available from the Census Bureau at the block or ZIP Code levels. You will apportion Pov65Up, the population aged 65 and older living in poverty, from block groups to noncoterminous ZIP Codes using the block-level SF1 attribute Age_65_UP as the indicator variable. So we are assuming that the poverty is uniformly distributed over the senior citizen population—clearly an approximation. Notice that you will not need any shapefiles of block groups for apportionment. This is because we have block centroids and polygons for location. Block groups are made up of blocks, and the 15-digit block identifier includes the block group identifier, BlkGrpID, in its first 12 digits. Normally, BlkGrpID is named STFID, but we renamed it here for clarity.

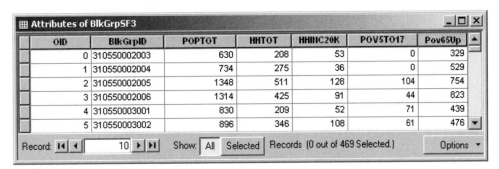

OID	BlkGrpID	POPTOT	HHTOT	HHINC20K	POV5TO17	Pov65Up
0	310550002003	630	208	53	0	329
1	310550002004	734	275	36	0	529
2	310550002005	1348	511	128	104	754
3	310550002006	1314	425	91	44	823
4	310550003001	830	209	52	71	439
5	310550003002	896	346	108	61	476

Record: 10   Show: All Selected   Records (0 out of 469 Selected.)   Options

ZipCodes.shp—Target set of polygons. Assuming that the GIS study being supported by apportionment is for Douglas County only, we clipped these ZIP Codes to correspond to Douglas County's boundary. Some of the original ZIP Code polygons spilled far over the county boundary.

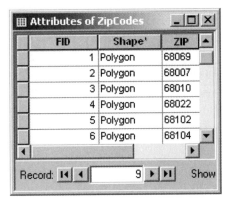

FID	Shape'	ZIP
1	Polygon	68069
2	Polygon	68007
3	Polygon	68010
4	Polygon	68022
5	Polygon	68102
6	Polygon	68104

Record: 9   Show

In the next map, the selected ZIP Codes and block groups are the ones that were clipped to the county boundary.

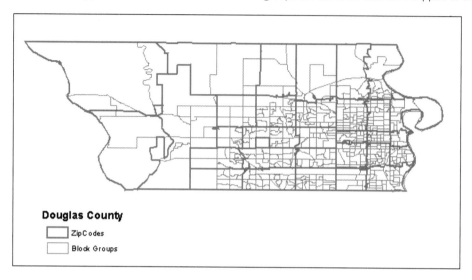

In the next map, you can see that the ZIP Code and block group polygons were obtained from different sources and digitized independently. Boundaries that in reality are shared do not match and have alignment problems. Also, many block groups, such as the one including the cursor, are split between two ZIP Codes.

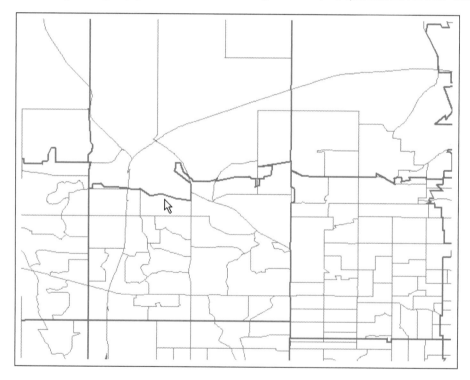

Blocks.shp—Polygon shapefile for census blocks. BlkID is the block identifier (generally named STFID, but here renamed for clarity), and AGE_65_UP is the SF1 census variable used as the indicator for apportionment.

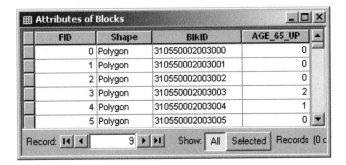

BlockCentroids.shp—Point shapefile for the centroids of census blocks.

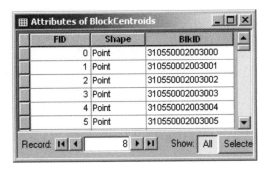

BlkGrpSF1.dbf—dBase table with the block-group level of data for the SF1 indicator, AGE_65_UP, and block group identifier, BlkGrpID. Each AGE_65_UP value here is the sum of many blocks from the attribute table of Blocks.shp and the denominator of a weight used in apportionment.

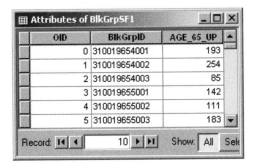

Spatially join ZipCodes to BlockCentroids

1 **Launch ArcMap and open Tutorial8-2.mxd from your \GistutorialHealth folder.**

2 **On the bottom of the table of contents, click the Source tab.**

ArcMap opens with all of the inputs to apportionment included: three shapefiles and two data tables.

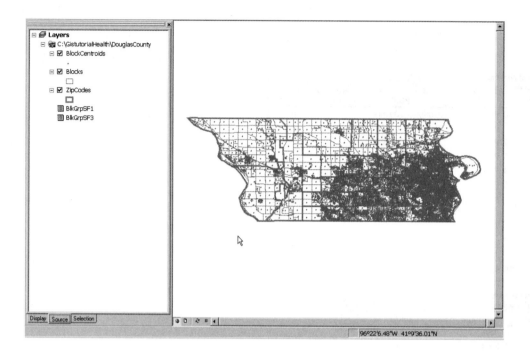

3 Click the ArcToolbox button.

4 In ArcToolbox, expand the Analysis Tools toolbox, then expand the Overlay toolset and double-click the Intersect tool.

5 In the Intersect dialog box, match the settings in the screen capture below.

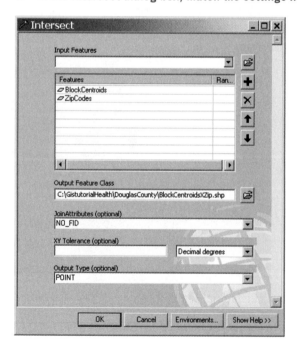

6 Click OK, then click Close.

Use the mid( ) function to calculate BlkGrpID

The new BlockCentroidsXZip shapefile needs the block group ID, so you will use the mid() function to create it from the BlkID field.

1   In the ArcToolbox panel, expand the Data Management Tools toolbox, then the Fields toolset. In the Fields toolset, double-click the Add Field tool.

2   In the Add Field dialog box, choose BlockCentroidsXZip from the Input Table drop-down list, in the Field Name box type **BlkGrpID**, choose TEXT from the Field Type drop-down list, and type **12** in the Field Length box.

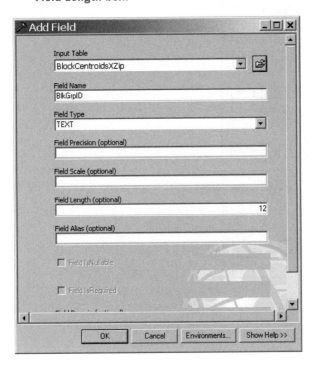

3   Click OK.

4   In the Fields toolset, double-click the Calculate Field tool.

5   In the Calculate Field dialog box, set the Input Table and Field Name settings to match the screen capture below, then click the Field Calculator button that's located just to the right of the Expression box.

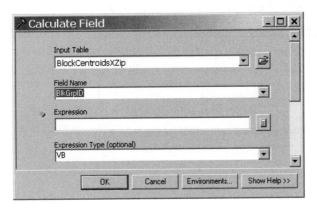

6   **Click the expression panel that's located in the lower half of the Field Calculator and type the
    following expression: mid([BlkID],1,12).**

This use of the mid( ) function extracts the first 12 characters of the text variable BlkID. The
first argument of the function is the name of the input text attribute, the second is an integer
giving the starting position for extraction, and the third is the number of characters to extract.

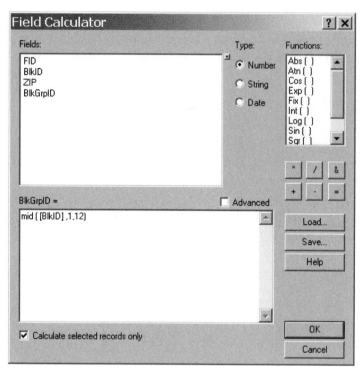

7   **Click OK in the two open dialog boxes.**

TURN

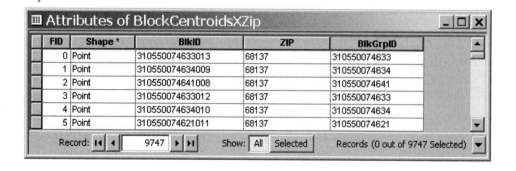

Open the BlockCentroidsXZip attribute table and verify that BlkGrpID is the first 12 digits of
BlkID. Notice how all of the blocks in the same block group have the same value for BlkGrpID.
Close the table.

Create a new field in BlockCentroidsXZip

Here you will create a new permanent field in BlockCentroidsXZip called Indicator. This field has the values of POP_65_UP that allows you to remove the join, which simplifies and speeds up later work.

1   In ArcToolbox, navigate to the Data Management Tools toolbox, Fields toolset, then double-click the Add Field tool.

2   In the Add Field dialog box, match the settings in the following screen capture.

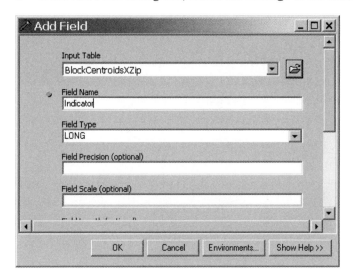

3   Click OK.

Join Blocks to BlockCentroidsXZip

Next, you need to join the block-level attribute, AGE_65_UP, to BlockCentroidsXZip.

1   In ArcToolbox, expand the Data Management Tools toolbox, then the Joins toolset. In the Joins toolset, double-click the Add Join tool.

2   In the Add Join dialog box, match the settings in the screen capture shown on the following page.

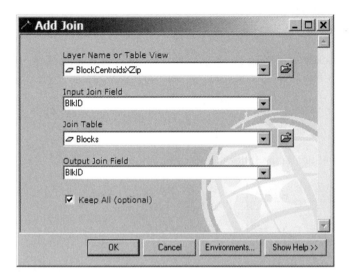

3   **Click OK and Close.**

Calculate new field

Next you will calculate the AGE_65_UP field from the Blocks attribute table to the BlockCentroidsXZip attribute table.

1   **In ArcToolbox, navigate to the Data Management Tools toolbox, Fields toolset, then double-click the Calculate Field tool.**

2   **Make the Input Table and Field Name settings as shown below, then click the Field Calculator button.**

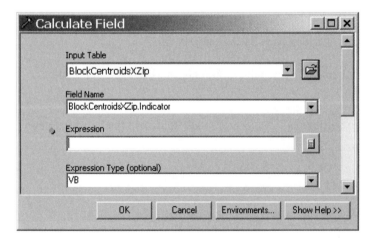

3   Enter the expression shown below.

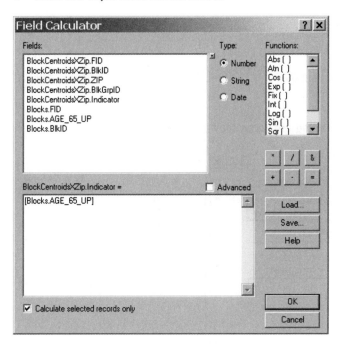

4   Click OK on the two open dialog boxes.

Remove Join

You no longer need the Blocks table, so you will remove the join here.

1   In ArcToolbox, navigate to the Data Management Tools toolbox, Joins toolset, then double-click the Remove Join tool.

2   In the Remove Join dialog box, match the settings shown in the screen capture.

3   Click OK.

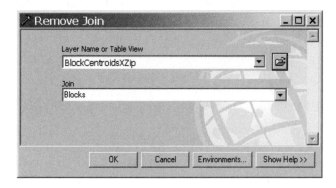

TURN

YOUR

Open the BlockCentroidsXZip attribute table to see the new values for the indicator field. These are the same as AGE_65_Plus.

Create another new field in BlockCentroidsXZip

Create another new attribute in BlockCentroidsXZip called IntID (meaning Intersection ID) that concatenates BlkGrpID with Zip.

1   In ArcToolbox, navigate to the Data Management Tools toolbox, Fields toolset, then double-click the Add Field tool.

2   In the Add Field dialog box, change the settings to those shown below.

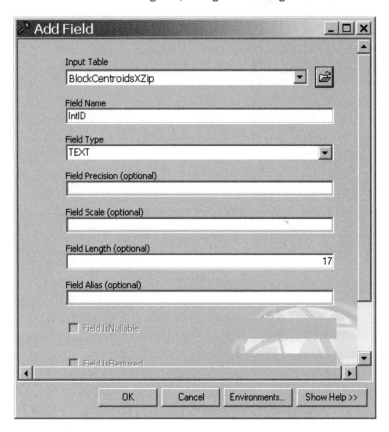

3   Click OK.

4   In the Joins toolset, click Add Join, then join the BlockCentroidsXZip and Blocks again.

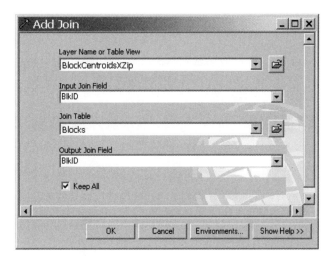

5   In the Fields toolset, double-click the Calculate Field tool.

6   In the Calculate Field dialog box, match the settings in the screen capture below, then click the Field Calculator button and create the expression currently shown in the Expression box below. Click OK.

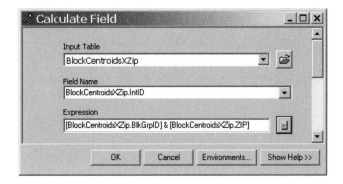

7   Click OK and Close.

TURN

YOUR

Remove the joined BlockCentroidsXZip and Blocks tables. Open the BlockCentroidsXZip attribute table and verify that it has attributes and values as seen below for the IntID field. If not, you will have to repeat some earlier steps to make corrections.

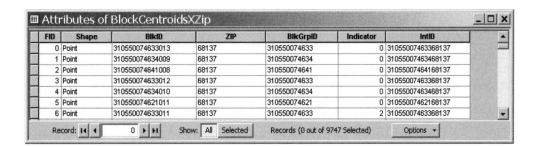

FID	Shape	BlkID	ZIP	BlkGrpID	Indicator	IntID
0	Point	310550074633013	68137	310550074633	0	31055007463368137
1	Point	310550074634009	68137	310550074634	0	31055007463468137
2	Point	310550074641008	68137	310550074641	0	31055007464168137
3	Point	310550074633012	68137	310550074633	0	31055007463368137
4	Point	310550074634010	68137	310550074634	0	31055007463468137
5	Point	310550074621011	68137	310550074621	0	31055007462168137
6	Point	310550074633011	68137	310550074633	2	31055007463368137

Record: |◄ ◄   0   ► ►| Show: All   Selected   Records (0 out of 9747 Selected)   Options ▾

Summarize Indicator field by IntID

The Indicator (AGE_65_UP) field can now be summed by the new IntID (BlockgroupID and ZIP) fields. Here you will aggregate (sum) the data using ArcToolbox tools. The dissolve tool has the capacity to sum, so that is what you will use. The result will be a new shape file of the aggregated data.

1   In the Data Management Tools toolbox, expand the Generalization toolset, then double-click the Dissolve tool.

2   In the Dissolve dialog box, match the settings shown in the following screen capture. Use the Statistics Field(s) drop-down list to populate the Field column located on the lower portion of the dialog box. Also, be sure to set the Statistic Type for each field by clicking the cell just to the right of the field name and choosing one of the statistic types.

Note: The Statistic Type FIRST is used because these are text fields.

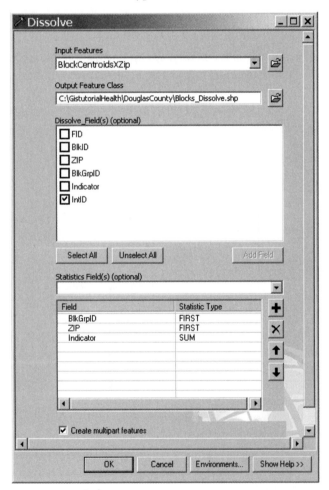

3   Click OK and Close.

YOUR TURN

Open the Blocks_Dissolve attribute table and examine its data. You will see that you have created useful data, although the dissolve tool has given strange names to the results. FIRST_BlkG contains the values that were in the original BlkGrpID field, FIRST_ZIP contains the original ZIP values. The SUM_Indica field contains the numerator of weights, which was generated from the sum of the AGE_65_Up field for each block group and ZIP Code-intersected polygon. Close the attribute table.

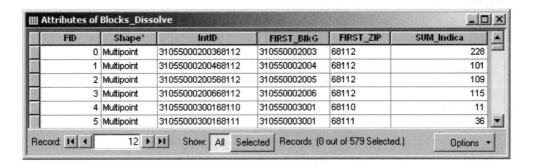

FID	Shape'	IntID	FIRST_BlkG	FIRST_ZIP	SUM_Indica
0	Multipoint	31055000200368112	310550002003	68112	228
1	Multipoint	31055000200468112	310550002004	68112	101
2	Multipoint	31055000200568112	310550002005	68112	109
3	Multipoint	31055000200668112	310550002006	68112	115
4	Multipoint	31055000300168110	310550003001	68110	11
5	Multipoint	31055000300168111	310550003001	68111	36

Record: 12   Show: All Selected   Records (0 out of 579 Selected.)   Options ▾

Add Denominator field

Next, you will add a field used as the denominator to calculate the weight of block groups within ZIP Codes.

1 **In the Data Management Tools toolbox, expand the Fields toolset, then double-click the Add Field tool.**

2 **In the Add Field dialog box, match the settings shown below.**

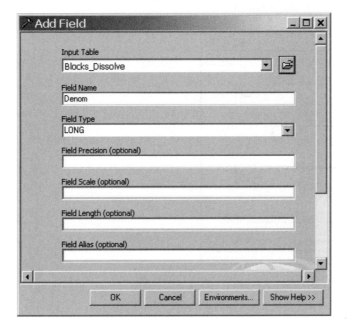

3 **Click OK.**

Join BlkGrpSF1 to Blocks_Dissolve

1   In the Data Management Tools toolbox, expand the Joins toolset, then double-click the Add Join tool.

2   In the Add Join dialog box, match the settings shown below.

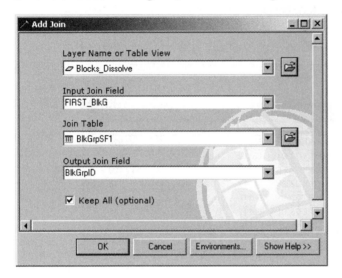

3   Click OK and Close.

Calculate Denominator field

1   Double-click the Calculate Field tool that's located in the Fields toolset.

2   In the Calculate Field dialog box, match the settings shown below.

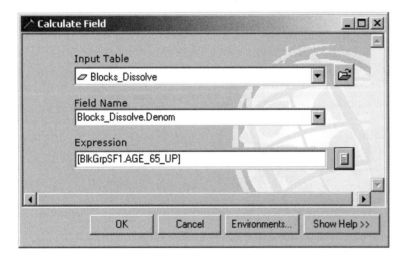

3   Click OK.

Remove the Join from Blocks_Dissolve

1   In the Data Management Tools toolbox, expand the Joins toolset, then double-click the Remove Join tool.

2   Make selections as follows.

(If you get an error icon for the Join field, click the list arrow and make the selection as shown.)

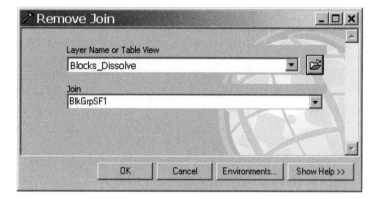

3   Click OK.

YOUR TURN

Examine the Blocks_Dissolve attribute table. The apportionment weights for the first four block groups—310550002003 through 310550002006—will all be 1 because those block groups are entirely inside ZIP Code 68112. Block group 31050003001, however, is split up between two ZIP Codes. Eleven out of 47 senior citizens (weight = 0.234) are in ZIP Code 68110 and the remaining 36 out of 47 (weight = 0.766) are in ZIP Code 68111. You will calculate these weights in the upcoming steps.

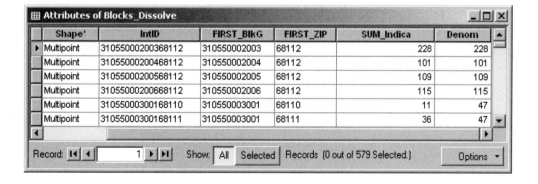

Shape*	IntID	FIRST_BlkG	FIRST_ZIP	SUM_Indica	Denom
Multipoint	31055000200368112	310550002003	68112	228	228
Multipoint	31055000200468112	310550002004	68112	101	101
Multipoint	31055000200568112	310550002005	68112	109	109
Multipoint	31055000200668112	310550002006	68112	115	115
Multipoint	31055000300168110	310550003001	68110	11	47
Multipoint	31055000300168111	310550003001	68111	36	47

Record: 1   Show: All Selected Records (0 out of 579 Selected.)   Options ▾

Calculate the apportionment weights

1 In the Data Management Tools toolbox, expand the Fields toolset, then double-click the Add Field tool.

2 In the Add Field dialog box, match the settings shown below.

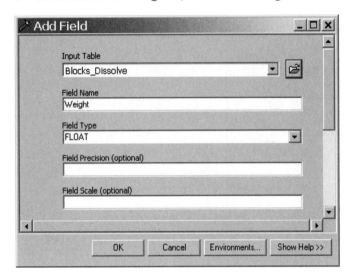

3 Click OK.

4 Double-click the Calculate Field tool.

5 In the Calculate Field dialog box, make the settings shown below. (Use the Field Calculator button to create the expression as follows.)

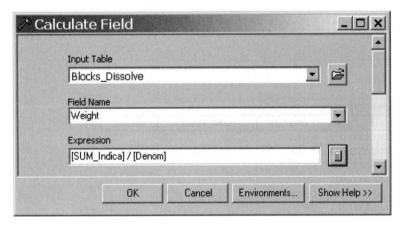

6 Click OK.

YOUR TURN

Open the Attributes of Blocks_Dissolve table and examine the weight field. A value of 1 means that the block group is entirely within a ZIP Code and a fraction means it is split between ZIP Codes. Close the attribute table.

Join and calculate SF3 poverty data to Blocks_Dissolve

Here you will calculate the poverty data for the elderly population based on the weighted values you just created.

1   In the Fields toolset, double-click the Add Field tool.

2   In the Add Field dialog box, match the settings shown below.

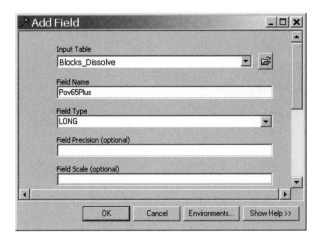

3   Click OK and Close.

4   In the Data Management Tools toolbox, expand the Joins toolset, then double-click the Add Join tool.

5   In the Add Join dialog box, match the settings shown below.

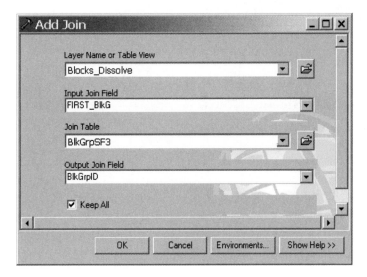

6   Click OK.

7   Double-click the Calculate Field tool.

8   In the Calculate Field dialog box, match the settings shown below.

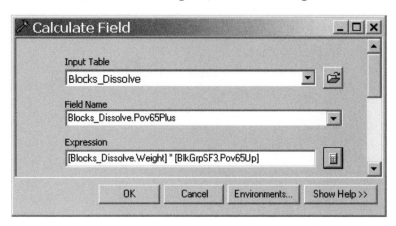

9   Click OK and Close.

TURN

YOUR

Examine the Blocks_Dissolve attribute table and compare it to the one below. We have used the shapefile's properties to turn off several irrelevant fields for ease of display. See how the weights have split up the SF3 value for block group 310550003001. Remove the current join between Blocks_Dissolve and BlkGrpSF3.

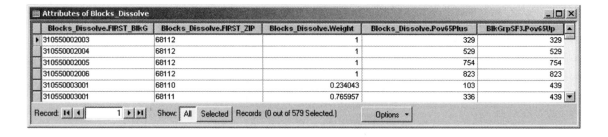

Blocks_Dissolve.FIRST_BlkG	Blocks_Dissolve.FIRST_ZIP	Blocks_Dissolve.Weight	Blocks_Dissolve.Pov65Plus	BlkGrpSF3.Pov65Up
310550002003	68112	1	329	329
310550002004	68112	1	529	529
310550002005	68112	1	754	754
310550002006	68112	1	823	823
310550003001	68110	0.234043	103	439
310550003001	68111	0.765957	336	439

Record: 1   Show: All Selected   Records (0 out of 579 Selected.)   Options ▾

Sum the SF3 attribute by ZIP Code

You can now aggregate the population over 65 living in poverty to ZIP Codes.

1   In the Data Management Tools toolbox, expand the Generalization toolset, then double-click the Dissolve tool.

2   In the Dissolve dialog box, match the settings shown below.

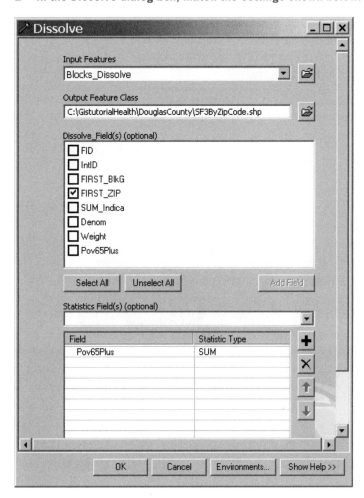

3   Click OK and Close.

Cleanup

1   Start Microsoft Excel and browse to your **\GistutorialHealth\DouglasCounty** folder and open **SF3ByZipCode.dbf**.

2   Change the name of the first column to Zip and the second to Pov65Up.

3 Right-click the column selector for column B and click Format, Cells, and Number; change the number of decimal places to 0; and click OK.

4 Click File, Save As, name the file **Pov65PByZip.xls** (Excel 97-2003 Workbook) and save it in your **\GistutorialHealth\DouglasCounty**.

YOUR TURN

Remove all layers except ZipCodes. Add Pov65PByZip.xls (Database) and join it to ZipCodes using the ZIP field. Create a choropleth map out of the ZipCodes layer using the Pov65Up field values. We used five classes and quantiles for the map below. When finished, save your project as \GistutorialHealth\Tutorial8-2.mxd and close ArcMap.

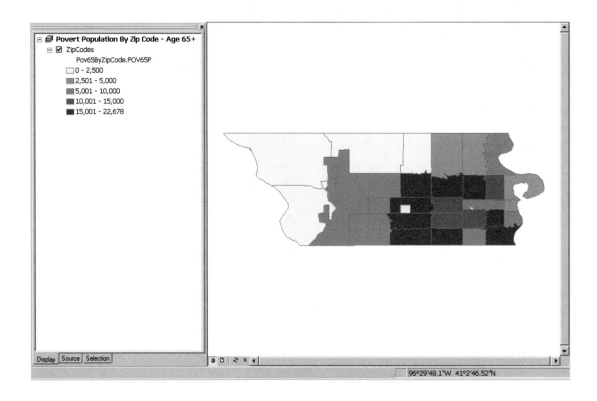

Start building a model

ArcToolbox includes a very modern and exciting graphical interface for creating workflow models. You do not need to know anything about programming to use this tool, just how to drag and drop graphical objects and fill out parameter forms for the objects, as you did throughout the previous apportionment section.

Create a new toolbox and model

1   Start ArcMap, open **Tutorial8-3.mxd** from your **\GistutorialHealth** folder, and click Open.

2   If necessary, open ArcToolbox.

3   Right-click anywhere inside the white area of ArcToolbox and click New Toolbox.

4   Change the name of the resulting toolbox to **Apportionment Tools**.

5   Right-click the new Apportionment Tools toolbox and click New, then Model.

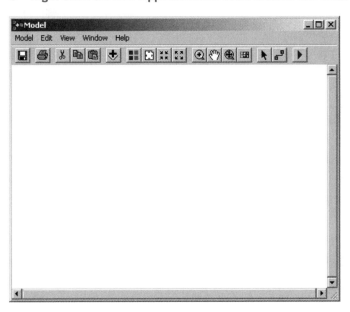

Spatially join ZIPCodes to BlockCentroids

All that is necessary to build the model is to repeat interactive steps, from the beginning of the apportionment section of this tutorial, in the context of a model.

1   From the ArcMap table of contents, click and drag BlockCentroids into the Model window.

2   Reposition the Model dialog box, the ArcMap table of contents, and ArcToolbox so you can see them all at the same time.

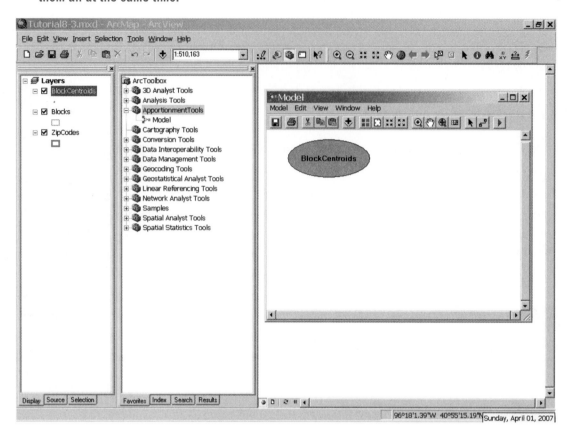

3   In ArcToolbox, expand the Analysis Tools toolbox, then the Overlay toolset.

4   Drag and drop the Intersect tool from ArcToolbox into the Model window, placing it just to the right of the BlockCentroids object.

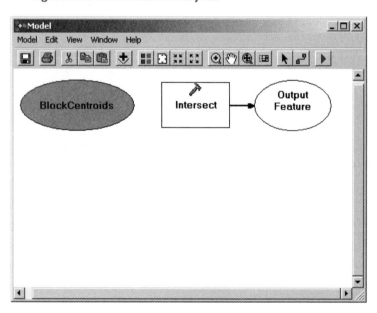

5   Click the Add Connection button 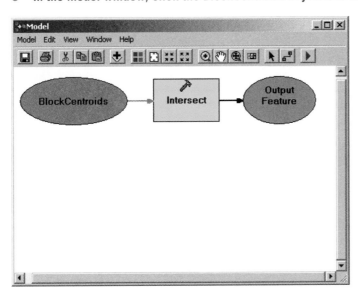 on the Model toolbar.

6   In the Model window, click the BlockCentroids object and drag a line to the Intersect object.

7   Double-click the Intersect object in the Model window, match the settings shown in the graphic below, then click OK.

Note: Name every shapefile, table, or field that you create with a digit 2 at the end to differentiate work here from the earlier interactive work.

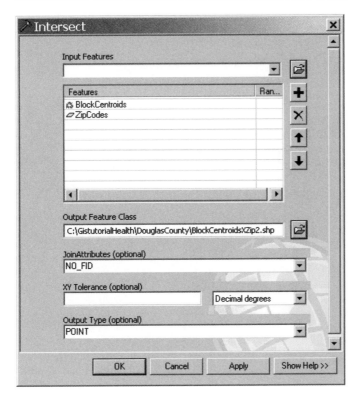

8   Click the pointer button [▲] on the Model toolbar.

9   Rearrange the objects as shown below.

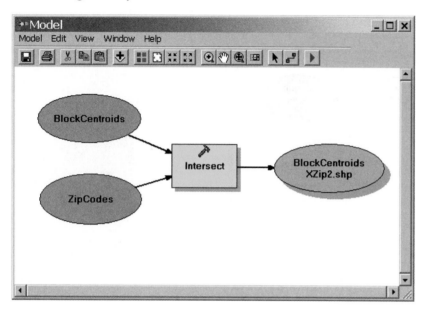

10 Click Model, Run Entire Model, and Close.

Add and calculate a field

1   In ArcToolbox, expand the Data Management Tools toolbox, then expand the Fields toolset.

2   From the Fields toolset, drag and drop the Add Field tool into the Model window.

3   Click the Add Connection button [⬚] on the Model toolbar.

4   Click the BlockCentroidsXZip2.shp object and drag a line to the Add Field object.

5   On the Model toolbar, click the pointer button.   [▲]

6   Double-click the Add Field object, then match the settings shown on the following page.

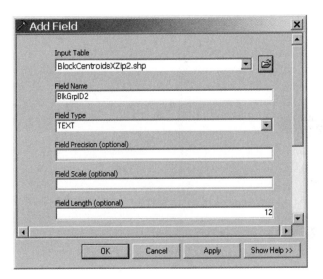

7   **Click OK.**

8   **Click the Add Field object in the Model window. Then, from the Model menu, click Model and then Run. Click Close when the process completes.**

The Run action, as opposed to Run Entire Model, runs only the selected object so that you can continue to try out your model, step by step, as you build it.

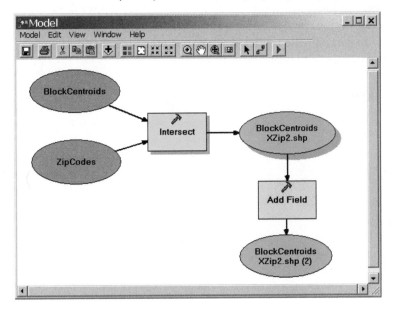

TURN

YOUR

Drag the Calculate Field tool to the model. Use BlockCentroidsXZip2.shp (2) object as the input to the Calculate Field Object and fill out the form to calculate BlkGrpID2 = mid([BlkID],1,12). Tidy up the appearance of your model. Run just the Calculate Field model.

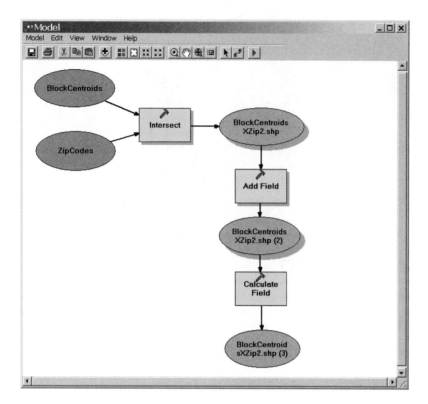

Using the model building tool, you can keep adding steps from the interactive ones done earlier in this tutorial until all of apportionment is carried out in the model. If you need to run the model in a new context, you can edit the model, open parameter forms, and make adjustments, such as changing the names of files or field names.

Summary

A common problem facing GIS analysts is that they obtain aggregate data for one set of polygons, but need to transform that data into a different set of polygons. In certain amenable cases, it's easy to make the transformation using simple data aggregation.

In other, more interesting cases, a good deal of work is needed to achieve an approximate solution. An example is U.S. Census 2000 Summary File 3 (SF3) data obtained from the Census 2000 long form. This data is available for census block groups and tracts, but not for very small census blocks or ZIP Codes. Much health-related data is available only by ZIP Codes, and while ZIP Codes do not have very good properties for analysis, they are all that is available. Thus, you need to transform SF3 data to ZIP Codes.

We call the corresponding approximation "apportionment" and use a Summary File 1 (SF1) census variable as an indicator variable. In this tutorial, we assumed that poverty is uniformly spread over the senior citizen population. So, we used the SF1 indicator variable for population age 65 or older as the indicator for the SF3 variable population age 65 or older living in poverty. The SF3 indicator variable is not available for the target polygons, but the SF1 indicator variable is.

You used ArcToolbox interactively to learn about and carry out apportionment. The benefit of using the tools, instead of the usual menu selections in ArcMap, is that they can be built into a macro or model, and reused in a single step. Automating this helps you apportion, and this tutorial helped you to start that process, which is easy to finish on your own.

EXERCISES

Exercise assignment 8-1

Population variables for health-service areas

Problem:

The health-referral areas that you examined in tutorial 8 are for studying health and health care across large areas of the country. Health-service areas are similar, except they are for state and local health-care market analysis. In this exercise, you will aggregate block-level populations to health-service areas in Nebraska and map the results.

Start with the following:

- **C:\GistutorialHealth\SolutionComponents\Chapter8\BlockCentroids.shp**—point shapefile of block centroids for Nebraska created from Nebraska blocks in tutorial 8.

- **C:\GistutorialHealth\Nebraska\NebraskaHSA.shp**—polygon shapefile of health-service areas in Nebraska.

Create a map comparing population in health-service areas

Begin a new project called C:\GistutorialHealth\Answers\Assignment8\Assignment8-1.mxd that includes a layout with choropleth maps comparing the total population, elderly population (over 65), young population (under 18), and households with single moms (FHH_CHILD) for Nebraska health-service areas.

Save new shapefiles to C:\GistutorialHealth\Answers\Assignment8.

Export your map to a PDF file called C:\GistutorialHealth\Answers\Assignment8\Assignment8-1.pdf.

Exercise assignment 8-2

Population in urban areas

Problem:

The study of health in urban versus rural settings is of particular interest as the nation faces a growing concern for health-care issues such as access to quality care. The Census Bureau defines "urban areas" to encompass densely settled areas that consist of census blocks with a population density of at least 1,000 people per square mile.

In this exercise, you will create census block centroids for Massachusetts and summarize these for urban areas to calculate the total, youth, and elderly populations for urban areas.

Start with the following:

- **C:\GistutorialHealth\Massachusetts\Outline.shp**—polygon shapefile of Massachusetts.

- **C:\GistutorialHealth\Massachusetts\CensusBlocks.shp**—polygon shapefile of Massachusetts census blocks.

- **C:\GistutorialHealth\Massachusetts\UrbanAreas.shp**—polygon shapefile of Massachusetts urban areas.

- **C:\GistutorialHealth\Massachusetts\MajorCities.shp**—point shapefile of major cities in Massachusetts for reference.

Create map aggregating and comparing populations in urban areas

Create a new project called C:\GistutorialHealth\Answers\Assignment8\Assignment8-2.mxd and add the above layers. Create point centroids for the census blocks and spatially join these to the urban areas to count the total population, young population (under 18), and elderly population (over 65) in the urban areas. Create a map layout comparing the total young and elderly populations normalized as a percentage to the total population in urban areas.

Save new shapefiles to C:\GistutorialHealth\Answers\Assignment8.

Export the map as a JPEG file called C:\GistutorialHealth\Answers\Assignment8\Assignment8-2.jpg.

What to turn in:

If you are working in a classroom setting with an instructor, you may be required to submit the exercises you created in chapter 8. Below are the files you are required to turn in. Be sure to use a compression program such as PKZIP or WinZip to include all files as one ZIP document for review and grading. Include your name and assignment number in the ZIP document <YourNameAssignment8.zip>.

ArcMap projects

C:\GistutorialHealth\Answers\Assignment8\Assignment8-1.mxd
C:\GistutorialHealth\Answers\Assignment8\Assignment8-2.mxd

New shapefiles

C:\GistutorialHealth\Answers\Assignment8\JoinedHSA_NebraskaCentroids.shp
C:\GistutorialHealth\Answers\Assignment8\MA_BlockCentroids.shp
C:\GistutorialHealth\Answers\Assignment8\JoinedUrbanAreas_MABlockCentroids.shp

Exported maps

C:\GistutorialHealth\Answers\Assignment8\Assignment8-1.pdf
C:\GistutorialHealth\Answers\Assignment8\Assignment8-2.jpg

OBJECTIVES

Examine raster basemap layers
Create a raster mask
Process a raster layer with mask
Create a hillshade raster layer
Make a kernel density map
Extract raster value points
Conduct a site suitability study
Build a model for risk index

GIS Tutorial 9

Using ArcGIS Spatial Analyst for demand estimation

This tutorial is an introduction to ArcGIS Spatial Analyst, an extension for ArcGIS Desktop. Spatial Analyst uses or creates raster datasets composed of grid cells to display data that is distributed continuously over space as a surface. In this tutorial, you will prepare and analyze a demand surface map for the location of heart defibrillators in the city of Pittsburgh with demand based on the number of out-of-hospital cardiac arrests with potential bystander help. You will also learn how to use Spatial Analyst's Raster Calculator to create a poverty index surface combining several census data measures from block and block-group polygon layers.

Health-care scenario

While most heart attacks occur in the home or in hospitals, approximately 20 percent occur in public places. Having automated defibrillators in public places is one innovation that increases the chances of victims surviving heart attacks. One study showed that defibrillators in public places saved twice as many heart attack victims as CPR by itself (*The Harvard Medical School Family Health Guide* 2008). As a result, health-care policy analysts in Pittsburgh, Pennsylvania, are working on a plan to provide defibrillators in some of Pittsburgh's public places. These analysts would like an estimate of demand or need for this emergency health service. They would also like to understand what factors contribute to heart attacks in public places: terrain, land use, socioeconomic condition, and so forth.

Available is a sample of heart attack incidences that have taken place in public over a five-year period in Pittsburgh. The sample was collected with the selection criterion that bystander help could be available, given the point locations of heart attacks. In addition, the policy analysts wish to add criteria that potential public defibrillator sites be in commercial areas as well as in peak areas for demand.

Solution approach

This study needs a large-scale analysis, down to the block level, to precisely determine where defibrillators should be located. Given address data for public-location heart attacks, it is certainly possible to geocode and map the corresponding points. Then it is possible to aggregate the points to counts per block and plot choropleth maps as an indication of demand for defibrillators in public locations. Pittsburgh, however, has 7,466 blocks. With that many areas, it becomes difficult to use vector graphics. For example, corresponding choropleth maps would have areas so small that it becomes impractical even to give polygons visible boundaries; there's little room left for color fill. The best treatment for polygons in this case is to plot their centroid points, symbolized with a color ramp to represent magnitudes such as number of heart attacks. That sort of map, however, is difficult to analyze visually and to process analytically.

Hence, you need a different type of map, one that deals with very small areas or continuously changing variables. Raster maps fill this need. They are rectangular arrays of very small, uniform, square cells analogous to pixels in an image file (such as JPEG or GIF format files). In addition to recording a value for each cell (such as heart attacks per unit area), raster maps store sufficient data to determine the geographic coordinates of each cell for plotting and display as background for vector map layers.

An additional problem with using choropleth maps to represent demand is that the data for each polygon is a sample and thus has sampling error. In other words, each block's displayed number of heart attacks should be thought of as an underlying mean value for that block plus a random error. Estimated mean demand is often a more reliable predictor of future demand than raw data because the random errors get averaged out. So, it would be better to use a mean surface for heart attacks than raw-data maps for predicting future demand.

The ArcGIS Spatial Analyst extension has the capacity to create and process raster maps in sophisticated ways. Key for this study is the density surface estimation capability, which uses data for polygon centroids as input and estimates mean surfaces as output in raster format. In particular, you will use kernel density estimation for producing a smoothed, mean surface for the number of heart attacks per square foot in Pittsburgh. With this output in hand, it is then possible to make multiple-criteria queries to identify potential locations for public defibrillators.

Raster graphics provide some unique GIS capabilities, some of which are needed in the current study. One is to easily combine data from different vector-based geographies. For example, in building a risk index for poverty, you will need to use block and block-group map layers as input. Both geographies are easily transformed to the same raster map cells via kernel density estimation. Then ArcGIS Spatial Analyst provides raster algebra and an interface to combine multiple raster inputs into a single index. You will use the innovative and well-reasoned approach of so-called "robust" or "improper" linear models (Dawes 1979). This kind of model combines two or more independent variables in a way that is predictive of a dependent variable when no dependent variable data is available. You will build a robust linear model for poverty, one of the determinants of heart attacks in public places.

The steps to building the robust model are many and complex. So instead of just following steps interactively, you will use ModelBuilder to build a stored macro that strings steps together into a single program that can be easily modified, reused, and communicated.

Examine raster basemap layers

You will start by opening a map document with both vector and raster map layers. The purpose of the maps that you will construct and analyze from the starting layers is to find areas suitable for locating public-access heart defibrillators to aid heart-attack victims. We obtained a sample of actual heart attack locations, which we geocoded as counts per census block centroid. We downloaded free base raster maps from U.S. Geological Survey (USGS) Web sites: http://seamless.usgs.gov/website/seamless/viewer.htm for digital elevation (a raster map called NED shaded relief, 1/3 arc second), and http://gisdata.usgs.net/website/MRLC/viewer.php for land use (a raster map called NLCD 2001). We also downloaded and preprocessed Census 2000 block and block-group maps and data, which you will use later in this chapter, from sites used in chapter 5.

Open a map document

1   Open ArcMap.

2   Click the An existing map radio button in the ArcMap window, and click OK.

3   Browse to the drive on which the **\GistutorialHealth** folder has been installed
     (e.g., C:\GistutorialHealth), select **Tutorial9-1.mxd**, and click Open.

The resulting map shows the digital elevation layer, named DEM, and the land-use layer with its downloaded file name, 28910720.tif. The DEM may look strange, but you will modify it and put it to good use later in this chapter. For the land-use layer, shades of red are developed areas and shades of green are forested areas (later you will see the full legend and a better view of the layer). Pittsburgh, of course, is the polygon for that municipality. The vector map layer called OHCA (out-of-hospital cardiac arrests) is the number of heart attacks over a five-year period per census block that occurred outside of hospitals where bystander help was possible because of location. Next, you will examine properties of the raster layers.

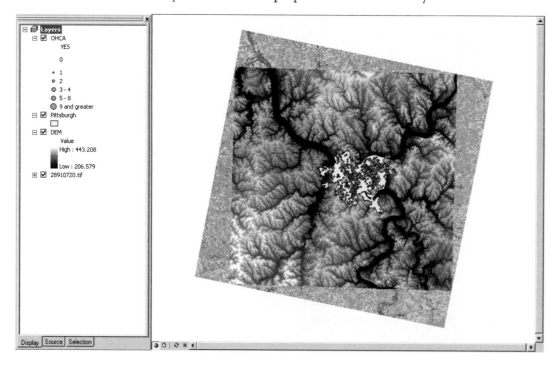

Examine raster map layer properties

1   In the table of contents, right-click **DEM** and click **Properties**.

2   Click the **Source** tab and scroll to the top of the window.

All raster maps are rectangular in their coordinate system. This one has 1,731 rows and 2,412 columns with square cells of 0.00027777778 decimal degrees on a side (10 meters at Pittsburgh's latitude). Each cell or pixel has a single value—elevation in meters—which is stored as a floating point number.

3   Scroll down until you see the **Extent** information.

Here you can see familiar-looking decimal degree values for the extent, so this layer is in geographic coordinates. ArcGIS projects it to the data frame's projection, state plane for southern Pennsylvania.

4   Scroll down further until you see the **Statistics** information.

These are statistics for elevation over the extent, including a mean elevation above sea level of 325.8 meters and maximum of 443.2 meters.

5   Close the **Layer Properties** window.

YOUR TURN

Examine the properties of 28910720.tif, the land-use layer. Notice that this is a projected layer, using a projection for the continental United States (and the reason why the layer tilts when ArcGIS projects it to the local, state plane projection). Also notice that the cell size is larger than that of DEM, 30 meters on a side, and that the values are integers corresponding to land-use categories. *Note: Rasters can only store floating point or integer values.*

Change raster attribute table size

Before you create raster masks, you need to increase the size of the raster attribute table (RAT). This value will be set for the remaining sections of this chapter.

1   Click **Tools, Options**.

2   Click the **Raster** tab, then the **Raster Attribute Table** tab and change the value to **100,000** as shown below.

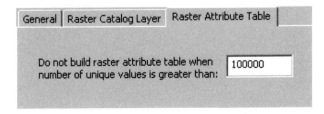

Create a raster mask

The site suitability study for locating defibrillators is for the city of Pittsburgh. While raster maps are rectangular, wouldn't it be good if you could display them just for the city and its irregular boundary? There's a way to accomplish this, by creating and using a mask for the Pittsburgh polygon. The mask is a raster map layer, and thus rectangular in shape, but it has the value "No Data" for cells outside of Pittsburgh, which ArcGIS displays using no color or clear. Thus, a mask uses a neat "trick" to enhance processing and display of raster maps to irregular boundaries.

1   Click the ArcToolbox button 🔲 and then drag the ArcToolbox window to the bottom of the table of contents to make more room in the map window.

2   In ArcToolbox, expand the Conversion Tools toolbox and then expand the To Raster toolset.

3   Double-click the Feature to Raster tool.

4   Click the Environments button at the bottom of the Feature To Raster window.

5   In the Environment Settings window, click General Settings, click the list arrow for Extent (scroll down if necessary), click Same as layer Pittsburgh, and click OK.

6   Make or type the following selections (assuming that your GistutorialHealth folder is on the C:\ drive):

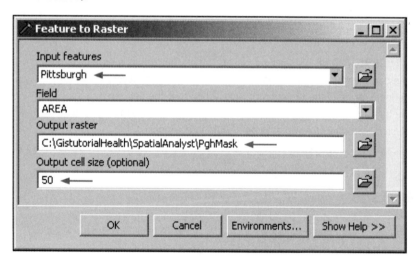

7   Click **OK** and then **Close** when the tool has finished processing.

8   In the table of contents, turn off the Pittsburgh vector layer.

9   Right-click **PghMask**, click **Properties**, and click the **Symbology** tab.

You can see in the lower right corner of the Symbology tab that NoData is set to display with no color. If you temporarily change the setting to any color, you will see the rectangular shape of the mask layer. You are now ready to create other raster layers that will display for Pittsburgh only, using the mask.

YOUR TURN

Note: You need to complete this task in order to do the next steps.

Add **PennHills.shp** to your map document from the **\GistutorialHealth\SpatialAnalyst** folder and zoom to that layer. Create a mask for Penn Hills Borough called PennHMask and save it in **\GistutorialHealth\SpatialAnalyst**. When finished, turn off the PennHills layers.

Hint: When you open the Feature to Raster tool, click the Environments button on that tool and change the extent to the PennHills layer and the cell size to 50.

10 Close the Properties window, turn off **PghMask**, and save your map document.

Process a raster layer with mask

ArcGIS can process and display a great many raster or image file formats. Its own file format is called ESRI grid. The land-use layer in your map document is a TIFF file format image as downloaded from the USGS site. To process it further, it's necessary to convert it to an ESRI grid. Then you can display it with PghMask.

Convert a TIFF image to a grid

1   Right-click the 28910720.tif layer in the table of contents and click Data, Export Data.

2   Make the selections shown in the following graphic.

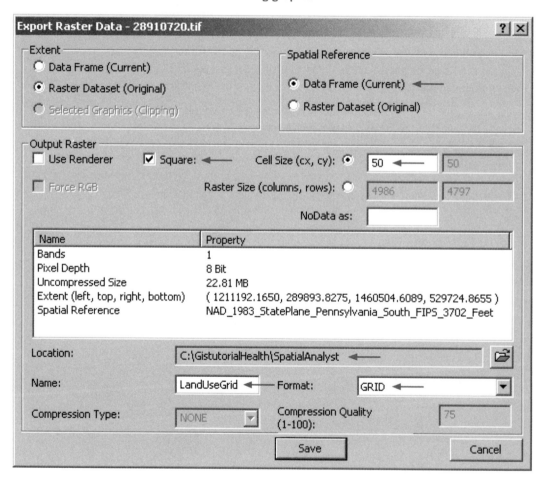

3   Click the Save button and then Yes.

4   In the table of contents, move the LandUseGrid layer to just below the OHCA layer.

Set ArcToolbox environment

Next, you need to set the environment for using the Spatial Analyst tools. Each time you use one of the tools, it automatically will use the environment settings, thereby saving you time.

1   **Click Tools, Extensions, check Spatial Analyst, and click Close.**

2   **In the ArcToolbox window, scroll to the top, right-click ArcToolbox and click Environments.**

3   **Click General Settings and set the environment as shown in the following graphic.**

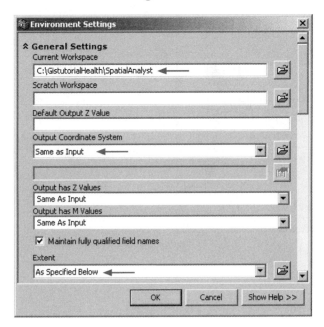

4   **Scroll down, click Raster Analysis Settings, and set the environment as shown in the following graphic.**

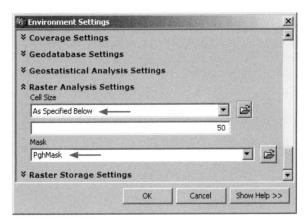

5   **Click OK.**

Extract land use using mask

Now the Spatial Analyst tools are ready for use in the environment that you set. One exception is that the Extract by Mask tool that you will use requires you to select the mask, even though it's already set in the environment.

1 **In ArcToolbox, expand Spatial Analyst Tools and then Extraction.**

2 **Double-click the Extract by Mask tool.**

3 **Fill out the tool as shown in the following graphic.**

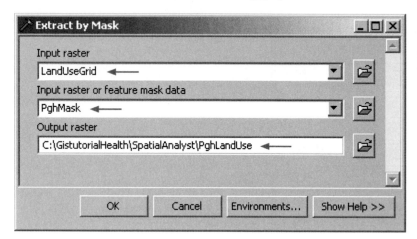

4 **Click OK, then Close.**

5 **In the table of contents, turn off the DEM, 28910720.tif, LandUseGrid, and PghLandUse layers.**

You will add a layer file next to correctly symbolize the new raster map.

6 **Click the Add Data button, browse to C:\GistutorialHealth\SpatialAnalyst, and double-click LandUsePgh.lyr.**

Note: If your data is *not* in C:\GistutorialHealth, you will have to open the layer's property sheet, click the Source tab, and set the source to the grid that you just created above, PghLandUse.

7   Right-click LandUsePgh and click Zoom to Layer.

The resulting map is much improved, following the outline of Pittsburgh. In the next section, you will make it even better by giving it a 3D appearance, using hillshade based on the DEM layer. As you might expect, the clusters of heart attack locations are in developed areas.

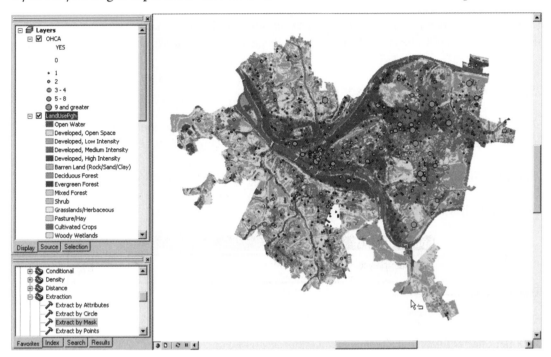

TURN

Using your PennHMask, extract LandUsePennH from LandUseGrid.

Hint: In the Extract by Mask tool, click the Environments button and set the General Settings extent and the Raster Analysis Settings mask to PennHMask. Be sure to make both settings!

Turn off your new layer, add **LandUsePgh.lyr** to your map document, change its source to LandUsePennH, and rename it **LandUsePennHills** in the table of contents.

When finished, turn off all of the Penn Hills layers and zoom back to the Pittsburgh layer if necessary.

Create a hillshade raster layer

The hillshade function simulates illumination of a surface from an artificial light source representing the sun. Two parameters of this function are the altitude of the light source above the surface's horizon in degrees and its angle (azimuth) relative to true north. The effect of hillshade to a surface, such as elevation above sea level, is striking, giving a 3D appearance due to light and shadow. You can enhance the display of another raster layer, such as land use, by making it partially transparent and placing hillshade beneath it. That's the objective of this section.

Add Spatial Analyst toolbar and set its options

Thus far, you have been using Spatial Analyst Tools in ArcToolbox to process raster layers. Sometimes it's more convenient or a better alternative to use the Spatial Analyst toolbar, which you will do next.

1 **Click View, Toolbars, scroll down if necessary, and click Spatial Analyst.**

The Spatial Analyst toolbar appears.

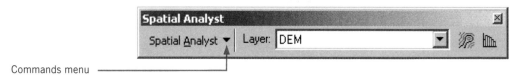

Commands menu

2 **Click the Spatial Analyst commands menu (see above) and click Options.**

3 **Click the General tab and enter the settings shown in the following graphic, where the working directory is C:\GistutorialHealth\SpatialAnalyst.**

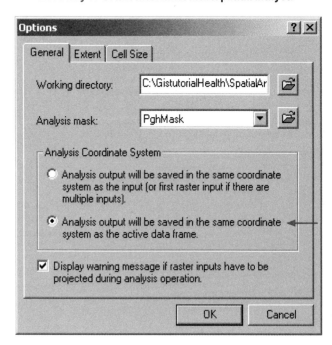

4 **Click the Extent tab and set the Analysis extent to Same as Layer "PghMask".**

Create hillshade for elevation

You will use the default values of the hillshade tool for azimuth and altitude. The sun for your map will be in the west (315°) at an elevation of 45° above the horizon.

1   On the Spatial Analyst toolbar, click the Spatial Analyst menu, then Surface Analysis, Hillshade.

2   Fill out the tool as shown in the following graphic.

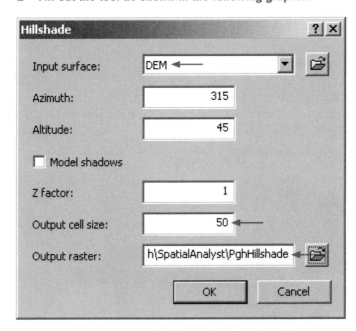

3   Click OK, then Yes.

Add contrast to hillshade

1   Right-click PghHillshade, click Properties, then the Symbology tab.

2   In the Stretch panel of the Color Ramp, click the Type drop-down arrow and choose Standard Deviations, in the n field type **3**, and click OK.

3   Move PghHillshade to just below LandUsePgh in the table of contents.

4   Right-click LandUsePgh in the table of contents, click Properties, then the Display tab.

5   Type **35** in the Transparency field and click OK.

That's the finished product. Heart attack locations are in some developed areas, but not all developed areas. Next, you will do additional spatial analysis on population statistics to see if you can determine a major factor affecting the incidence of heart attacks.

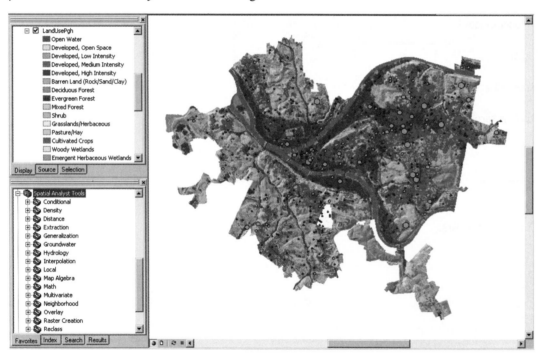

YOUR TURN

Create PennHshade and display it under a 35% transparent LandUsePennHills.

Hint: Change the Options in the Spatial Analyst toolbar so that the Analysis mask is PennHMask and extent is PennHMask.

When finished, save your map document.

Make a kernel density map

The incidence of myocardial infarction (heart attacks) outside of hospitals in the United States for ages 35 to 74 is approximately 5.6 per thousand males per year and 4.2 per thousand females per year (Rosamond, et al. 1998). You will use a point shapefile of census block centroids in Allegheny County to calculate the expected number of heart attacks based on incidence. For convenience, this expected value is also called incidence. The attribute table of this shapefile has the incidence attribute already calculated, Inc = [Fem35T74] × 0.0042 + [Male35T74] × 0.0056, where Fem35T74 is the population by block of females age 34 to 74, and Male35T74 is the corresponding population for males. The question is whether incidence does a good job of estimating the observed heart attacks in the OHCA point file.

Open a map document and examine environmental settings

The map document that you will open shows the observed locations of heart attacks (outside of hospitals and with the potential of bystander assistance), block centroids symbolized with a color gradient for heart attack incidence, and other supporting layers.

1   In ArcMap, open **Tutorial9-2.mxd** from the **\GistutorialHealth** folder.

The cartographic treatment for block centroids is as good as possible using point markers, but is somewhat difficult to interpret. Another representation for incidence is obtained by estimating the smoothed mean of the spatial distribution using a method such as kernel density smoothing. This method estimates the incidence as heart attacks per unit area (density) and has two parameters: cell size and search radius. There's no "science" of how to set these parameters, but the larger the search radius, the smoother the estimated distribution. When smoothing a particular cell, the farther away (up to the search radius), the less influence that other points have. Read ArcGIS Desktop Help for Kernel Density Smoothing to learn more about this method.

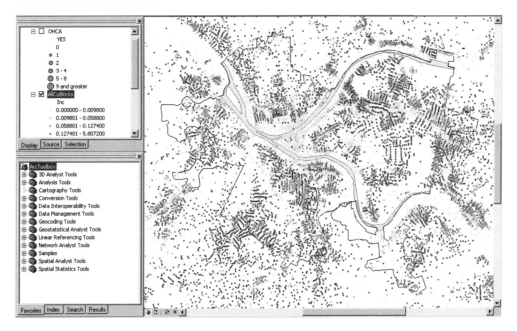

YOUR TURN

Tutorial9-2.mxd has the environmental settings for ArcToolbox and the Spatial Analyst toolbar already set. Examine the settings for both.

Note: If you used a path other than C:\GistutorialHealth\SpatialAnalyst for your files, you will have to reset the workspace location for environments.

Optional: Using Select by Location, select all block centroids completely within Pittsburgh, open the attribute table of AllcoBlocks, right-click the Inc column, select Statistics, and note the sum (684 for Pittsburgh). That's the expected annual number of heart attacks in Pittsburgh outside of hospitals. You will check that number to see if the smoothed density surface is correct. Clear selections and close the attribute table.

Make a density map for heart attack incidence

The OHCA map layer shows heart attacks per census block in Pittsburgh. Blocks in Pittsburgh average a little less than 300 feet per side in length. Suppose that policy analysts estimate that a defibrillator with public access can be made known to residents and retrieved for use as far away as 2.5 blocks from the location (on average, the middle of a block segment). They thus recommend looking at areas that are five blocks by five blocks in size, or 1,500 feet on a side, with defibrillators located in the center. Therefore, you will start out with a 150-foot cell and 1,500-foot search radius.

1 From the Spatial Analyst menu, click Density.

2 Make the selections shown in the following graphic.

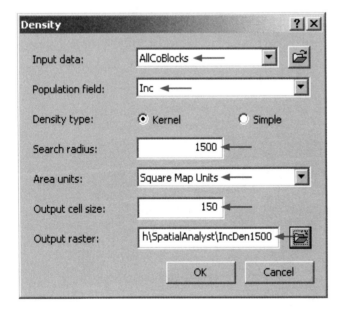

3 Click OK.

4   Right-click IncDen1500, click Properties, the Symbology tab, Yes, and the Classify button.

5   Click the drop-down list for Classification Method and choose Standard Deviation.

Standard Deviation is a good option for showing variation in raster grids. You control the number of categories in the next step by choosing the fraction of standard deviation for which to create break points, every 1, 1/3, 1/4, etc., standard deviations.

6   Click the drop-down list for Interval size, choose 1/3 Std Dev, and click OK.

7   Select the color ramp that runs from green to yellow to red, and click OK.

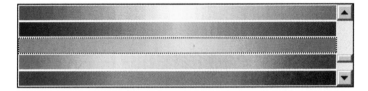

8   Turn on the OHCA layer and turn off AllCoBlocks.

Incidence appears to do a good job of matching clusters of the OHCA heart attack data in many, but not all areas. For example, there's a cluster in Pittsburgh's central business district (triangle just to the right of where the three rivers join), but estimated incidence is low there. The problem is that the density map, based on population data and incidence rates, shows expected heart attacks per square foot in reference to where people live, not necessarily where they have heart attacks. Many people shop or work in the central business district, but few live there.

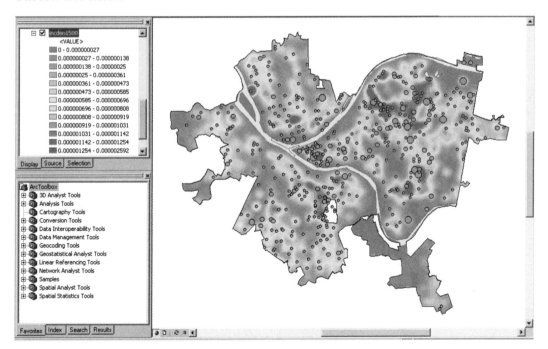

YOUR TURN

Check the density surface, to see if it makes sense. The estimated incidence that you found using block centroids was 684. Open the properties sheet for the density surface, click the Symbology tab, and click Classify. There you will find useful statistics: 72,315 cells with a mean of 0.000000417 heart attacks per square foot. Remember that each cell is 150 feet by 150 feet. You should find that this corresponds to a total of 679 heart attacks (a slightly more precise estimate of the mean from the Source tab, 0.0000004204, yields exactly 684). So what kernel density smoothing did was to move the input number and locations of heart attacks around, to distribute them smoothly. The result is a better estimate of incidence than raw data, because smoothing averages out randomness.

YOUR TURN AGAIN

Create a second kernel density surface for incidence, called IncDen3000, with all inputs and outputs the same except use a search radius of 3,000 instead of 1,500. Symbolize the output the same as IncDen1500. While keeping IncDen1500 turned on, turn IncDen3000 on and off to see the differences in the two layers. IncDen3000 is more spread out, smoother, but it has the same corresponding number of estimated heart attacks, 684.

Extract raster value points

While the estimated densities appear to match the actual heart attack data in OHCA, the match may or may not stand up to closer investigation. ArcToolbox has a tool that will extract point estimates from the raster surface for each point in OHCA. Then you can use the extracted densities multiplied by block areas to estimate number of heart attacks. If there is a strong correlation between the estimated and actual heart attacks, there would be evidence that population alone is a good predictor of heart attacks.

1   In ArcToolbox, expand Spatial Analyst Tools and the Extraction toolset.

2   Double-click the Extract Values to Points tool.

3   Make the selections shown in the following graphic.

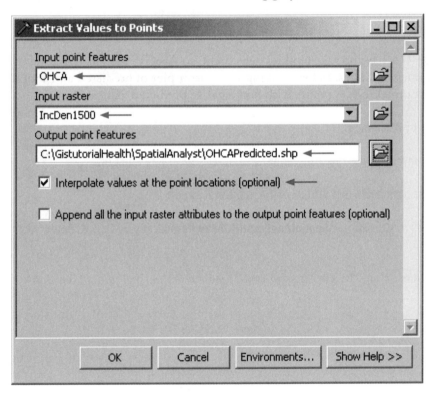

4   Click OK, then Close.

The resultant layer, OHCAPredicted.shp, has an attribute, RASTERVALU, which is an estimate of heart attack density, or heart attacks per square foot, in the vicinity of each block.

Calculate predicted heart attacks

You can expect that the resultant estimate will be larger than the actual number of heart attacks in OHCA's YES attribute, which just has heart attacks in which bystander help could have been available, given the location.

1   Right-click OHCAPredicted and open its attribute table.

2   Click Options, Add Field, and add a field called **Predicted** that will contain Float data values.

3   Right-click the Predicted column heading and click Field Calculator, Yes.

4   Create the expression 5 * [RASTERVALU] * [AREA], and click OK.

OHCA data is a five-year sample for heart attacks, thus the expression includes the multiple 5.

5   Close the attribute table.

A few of the points in OHCA have no raster values near them, so ArcGIS assigns the value -9999 to them to signify missing values. Before looking at a scatter plot of predicted and actual values, you will first select only OHCA points with nonnegative predicted values.

6   Click Selection, Select by Attributes.

7   For the OHCAPredicted layer, create the expression "Predicted" >= 0 and click OK.

8   In the table of contents, right-click OHCAPredicted, click Data, Export Data.

9   Export selected features to **\Gistutorial\SpatialAnalyst\OHCAPredicted2.shp** and click Yes to add the shapefile to the map.

10 Clear the selected features, close the Attributes of OHCA Predicted table, and turn off the OHCA_ Predicted layer.

Create a scatter plot of actual versus predicted heart attacks

Note: While Pittsburgh has a total of 7,466 blocks, only 1,509 blocks had heart attacks. The scatter plot that you will eventually construct includes data only for the 1,509 blocks, but should ideally include the balance of the total blocks, which had actual values of zero but predicted values sometimes much larger than zero. Nevertheless, you will be able to get an indication of the correlation between predicted and actual heart attacks. Adding the balance of blocks would make the correlation worse, but the correlation is actually already very low, as you will see next.

1   **Click Tools, Graphs, Create.**

2   **Make the selections shown in the following graphic.**

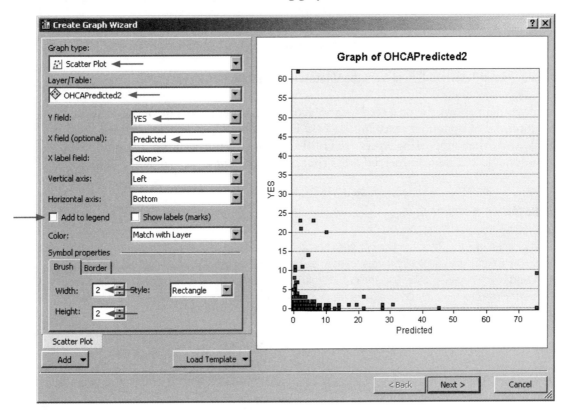

3   **Click Next, Finish.**

At the scale of blocks, evidently the predicted values correlate poorly with the actual values. If you export the corresponding data to a statistical package or Microsoft Excel, you can find that the correlation coefficient between predicted and actual values is only 0.0899, which is very low. Evidently, factors other than where the population resides affects the locations and clustering of heart attacks occurring outside of hospitals.

4   **Save your map document.**

Conduct a site suitability study

It seems that the location of heart attacks within Pittsburgh may have several determining factors in addition to population distribution. The strategy for finding suitable sites for locations of heart defibrillators should thus directly use the available data on heart attacks by census block to create an expected demand surface, and then apply several criteria to the surface. Kernel density smoothing of the heart attack data removed randomness from the spatial distribution, thereby providing a more reliable estimate of demand. Criteria include that there should be commercial land uses in the vicinity of heart attack clusters for the location of defibrillators and that there be a high enough number of heart attacks to warrant defibrillators.

Open a map document

The map document you will open has vector map layers you will convert to raster layers for site suitability queries.

1   In ArcMap, open **Tutorial9-3.mxd** from the **\GistutorialHealth** folder.

The map document shows the observed locations of heart attacks (outside of hospitals and with the potential of bystander assistance), a 600-foot buffer of commercially zoned areas in Pittsburgh, and other supporting layers. The 600-foot (or two-block) buffer of commercial areas includes adjacent noncommercial areas that have sufficient access to defibrillators.

Convert buffer to a raster layer

The ZoningCommercialBuffer layer has two polygons and corresponding records with a single attribute, Commercial. The Commercial value of 1 corresponds to commercial land use or land within 600 feet of commercial land use. The other value, 0, is the balance of Pittsburgh and includes all other zoned land uses. You will convert this vector layer into a raster layer using a conversion tool. First, however, you need to select both records in the vector file for them to convert.

1   Right-click the ZoningCommercialBuffer layer and click Open Attribute table.

2   Select both records by clicking the small gray box to the left of the first row, then dragging the mouse so both rows are highlighted.

3   Close the table.

4   In ArcToolbox, expand the Conversion toolbox and then the To Raster toolset.

5   Double-click the Feature to Raster tool.

6   Click the Environments button at the bottom of the Feature to Raster window, click the Raster Analysis Settings category, click the drop-down for Cell Size, select As Specified Below, set the cell size to 50, and click OK.

7   Make the selections shown in the following graphic.

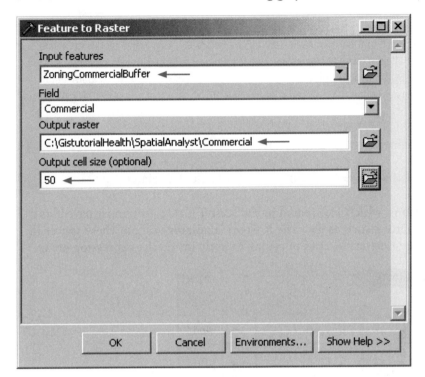

8   **Click OK, then Close.**

9   **Turn off the ZoningCommercialBuffer layer, right-click Commercial, click Properties, click the Symbology tab, in the left Show panel click Unique Values, click Yes (to compute unique values), and resymbolize the new Commercial area to have two colors: white for noncommercial (value 0) and gray for commercial (value 1).**

YOUR TURN

Note: You need to complete this task in order to do the next steps.

Create a kernel density map based on the YES attribute of the OHCA that has 150-foot cells and a search radius of 1,500 feet. Call the new raster layer **HeartAttack**. Symbolize the layer using the standard deviation method with interval size 1/3 Std Dev. Use the green to yellow to red color ramp. Turn off the OHCA layer.

Calculate a simple query

First, you will query your kernel density map, HeartAttack, for areas that have sufficiently high heart attack density to merit a defibrillator. Suppose that policy makers seek 25-block areas, roughly five blocks on a side, that would have 10 or more heart attacks every five years in locations where bystander help is possible. A square 25-block area is 5×300 feet = 1,500 feet on a side with 1,500 feet $\times$ 1,500 feet = 2.25×10^6 square feet of area. Thus, the heart attack density sought is 10 heart attacks / 2.25×10^6 square feet = 0.000004444 heart attacks per square foot or higher.

1   **From the Spatial Analyst menu, click Raster Calculator.**

2   **Create the expression [HeartAttack] >= 0.00000444 in the Raster Calculator.**

Note: Map algebra expressions, which are created in the Raster Calculator, must have blank spaces on both sides of operators, such as >=. The Raster Calculator will put these spaces in for you if you click its keypad buttons instead of typing directly inside the expression area.

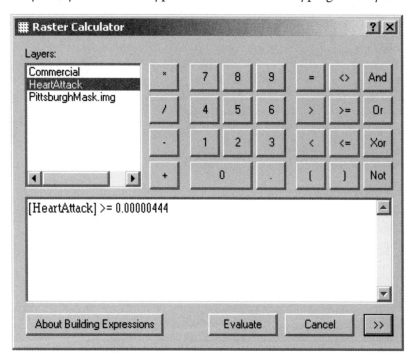

3   **Click Evaluate.**

ArcGIS creates a temporary raster layer called Calculation that has the results. There are two values: 0 is the value for cells that do not satisfy the criterion and 1 is for cells that do.

4 Resymbolize Calculation so that 0 has no color and 1 is dark blue, and make sure that HeartAttack is turned on and below Calculation.

You can see that relatively few peak areas, eight, have sufficiently high heart attack density. Some of them are likely too small in area, but you will not make that determination until all query criteria have been considered.

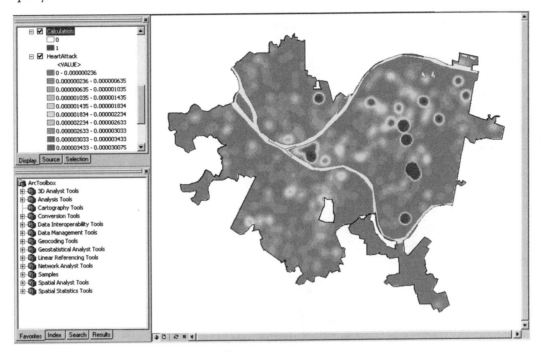

Calculate a compound query

Next, you will include a second criterion—locations within the commercial buffer—in the query for suitable defibrillator sites. You simply need to add the second criterion with an "AND" connector.

1 **From the Spatial Analyst menu, click Raster Calculator.**

2 **Create the expression [HeartAttack] >= 0.00000444 & [Commercial] == 1.**

Note: The "equals" operator is "==".

3 **Click Evaluate.**

ArcGIS creates a second temporary raster layer called Calculation2 that has the results.

4 **Resymbolize Calculation2 so that 0 has no color and 1 is light blue and make sure that Calculation and HeartAttack are turned on and below Calculation2.**

As you would expect, adding a second criterion with the AND connector has reduced the size of areas meeting criteria. Three of the formerly promising areas have been significantly reduced.

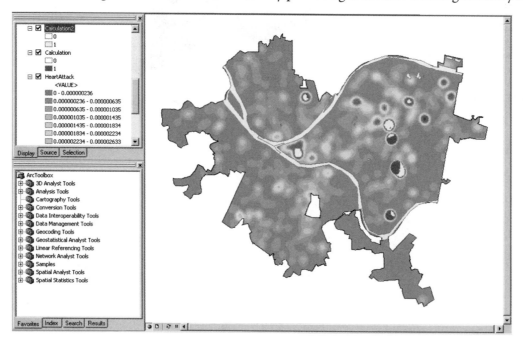

YOUR TURN

Turn on the Streets layer and zoom to each feasible area to check the third criterion that there be at least 25 blocks, or 2.25 million square feet, roughly in a square area. Use the Measure tool on the toolbar to measure feasible areas. Which areas remain feasible? What would you report back to policy makers?

5 **Save the map document.**

Build a model for risk index

Another variable that may be predictive of heart attacks is poverty. People who live in poverty often have poor health care, an unhealthy diet, and unhealthy habits such as smoking—all factors leading to higher incidence of heart attacks.

Often analysts wish to combine several map layers to yield a single, composite layer. For example, one study suggests that the following census variables are all indicative of poverty: (1) population below the poverty income line, (2) female-headed households with children, (3) population with less than a high school education, and (4) workforce males who are unemployed (O'Hare and Mather 2003).

A simple method for combining such measures into a poverty index, attributed to Robyn Dawes, is called an "improper" or unweighted linear model (Dawes 1979). If you have a reasonably good theory that several variables are indicative or predictive of a dependent variable of interest (and whether the dependent variable can be directly observed or not), then Dawes makes a good case that all you need to do is to remove scale from each input, so each has the same weight, and then average the scaled inputs to create a predictive index.

In this section, you will create an improper linear model for poverty by calculating Z-score values (data scaled by subtracting the mean and dividing by the standard deviation) for the above-mentioned variables and averaging them. The process of building the index is complex and error-prone, so you will use ArcGIS's ModelBuilder to string ArcToolbox tools together and make the process easy and more error proof.

Open a map document

The map document you are about to open has the two needed inputs for preparing a poverty index, AllCoBlkGrps.shp, which has block group centroids and needed attributes (NoHighSch2 = population with less than high school education, Male16Unem = males in the workforce who are unemployed, and Poverty = population below poverty income), and AllCoBlocks.shp, which has block centroids and the attribute FHH = female headed households with children. The attributes listed above for block groups are not available at the smaller and thus more desirable block level, so your study will have to use data from both geographies.

1   In ArcMap, open **Tutorial9-4.mxd** from the **\GistutorialHealth** folder.

Shown are the block group centroids and block centroids, each displaying one of the four poverty indicators via a color ramp. You can see that it is difficult to represent the spatial patterns effectively using vector graphics, plus it is difficult to integrate the information from two spatial distributions. The raster index that you will create will do a better job on both issues.

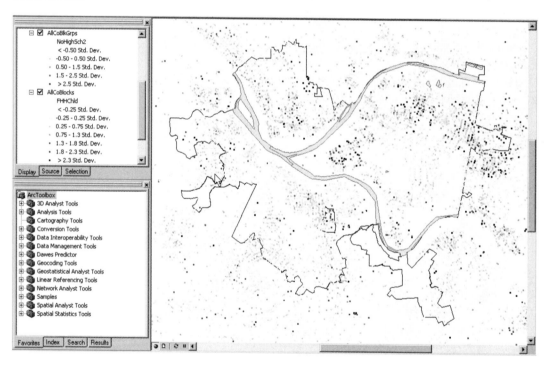

Create a new toolbox and model

You will create a model for producing a poverty index that will store every step, making the end result a reusable macro.

1 Click Tools, Options, then click the Geoprocessing tab, browse to **\GistutorialHealth \SpatialAnalyst\Toolboxes** to set the My Toolboxes folder, and click OK.

2 Right-click the ArcToolbox window and click New Toolbox.

3 Rename the new toolbox Unweighted Indices.

4 Right-click the new Unweighted Indices toolbox, then click New, Model.

The ModelBuilder window opens where you will create the poverty index model.

5 Click Model, Model Properties. On the General tab, for Name type **PovertyIndex** (no spaces allowed) and for Label type **Poverty Index**. You do not need to enter a description. Click OK.

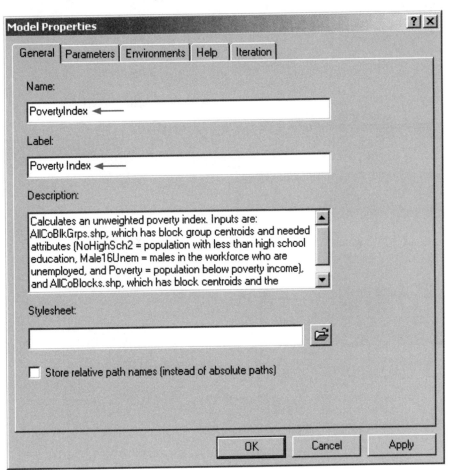

Create a kernel density layer for an input

The first step is to create kernel density layers for the four inputs. After you create model elements for one kernel density layer, you can easily copy them and make adjustments for the remaining three.

1   In ArcToolbox, expand Spatial Analyst Tools and then Density.

2   Drag the Kernel Density tool into the model.

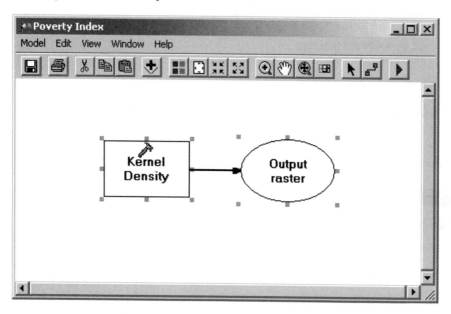

3   In the model, right-click Kernel Density and click Open.

4   Type or make the selections as shown in the following graphic.

Note: The Area units field is grayed out at first, but becomes available after you select AllCoBlocks as the input layer.

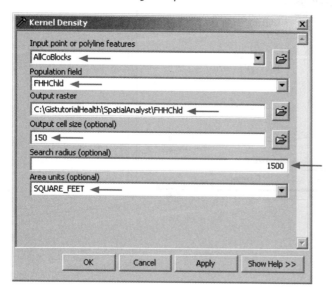

5   Click OK.

The tool does not run, but its settings are saved. You'll run the tool later.

6   Right-click the Kernel Density tool element, click Rename, and change the name to **FHHChld Kernel Density.**

You can click individual elements and resize them to make labels more readable.

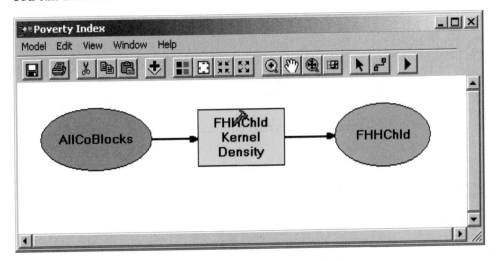

7   Right-click FHHChld Kernel Density, click Run, then Close.

8   Add the new FHHChld raster layer to the map document by right-clicking the FHHChld element and clicking Add to Display. Resymbolize the new layer to your liking, using the Classified method.

9   Turn off the AllCoBlkGrps and AllCoBlocks layers.

Note: If you have to close your map document and need to reopen and work on it later, you will have to open the Poverty Index model. In ArcToolbox, expand Unweighted Indices, right-click Poverty Index, and click Edit. Your model window will open.

Create a kernel density layer for a second input

You can reuse the model elements you just built. While blocks work very well with a search radius of 1,500 feet, there are fewer block groups (and the remaining three poverty inputs are at the block-group level), so a larger search radius of 3,000 feet is needed for them.

1   In the Model window, right-click FHHChld Kernel Density and click Copy.

2   Click Edit, Paste.

3   Right-click the new FHHChld Kernel Density 2 model element and rename it **NoHighSch Kernel Density.**

4   Right-click NoHighSch Kernel Density and click Open.

Ignore the error messages. You will make changes that eliminate them.

5   Type or make the selections shown below.

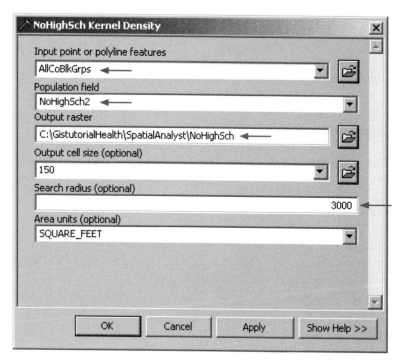

6   Click OK.

7   Right-click FHHChld(2) and rename it **NoHighSch.**

8   Right-click NoHighSch Kernel Density, click Run, and then Close.

9   Add NoHighSch to your map document and resymbolize it to your liking, using the Classified method.

10 Save your model.

YOUR TURN

Note: You must do this task in order to complete the exercise.

Copy and paste the NoHighSch Kernel Density model element two times to use block group attributes Male16Unem and Poverty to create two new raster layers of the same names. Then run each of the two new model elements and add the new raster maps and resymbolize them. Examine each of the four raster maps. You will see that they have overlapping but different patterns. The index will combine these patterns into a single, overall pattern. Save your model.

Your model should look like the following graphic. If your output names are different, you won't be able to run the raster calculation in the next step.

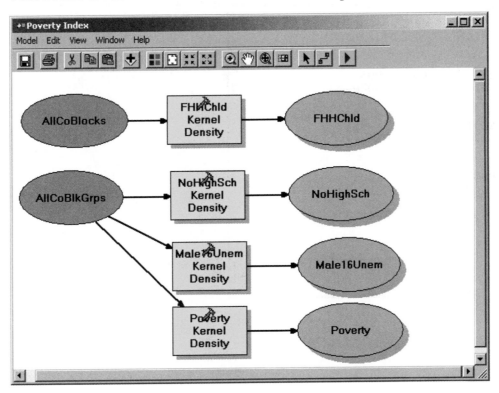

Note: The inputs can be made parameters, allowing the model to be reused for any geographic area in which you want to calculate the same census variables.

YOUR TURN

Before you can perform the analysis calculation in the next step, you need to collect some data; namely, the mean and standard deviation of each layer you just created. You can get these statistics by opening each layer's Source property sheet, then copying and pasting them to a word-processing file; you will then be able to easily copy and paste them into the Raster Calculator to avoid extensive typing. For a shortcut, a copy of the desired file is in **\Gistutorial \SpatialAnalyst\Statisics.txt**, as described in the next step.

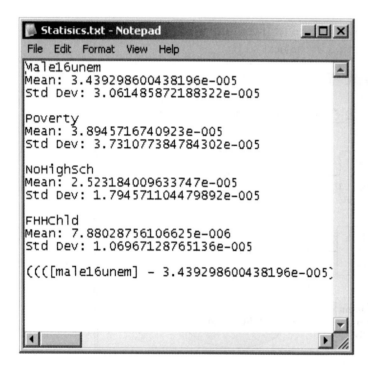

```
Statisics.txt - Notepad                          _ □ x
File  Edit  Format  View  Help
Male16unem
Mean: 3.439298600438196e-005
Std Dev: 3.061485872188322e-005

Poverty
Mean: 3.8945716740923e-005
Std Dev: 3.731077384784302e-005

NoHighSch
Mean: 2.523184009633747e-005
Std Dev: 1.794571104479892e-005

FHHChld
Mean: 7.88028756106625e-006
Std Dev: 1.06967128765136e-005

((([male16unem] - 3.439298600438196e-005)
```

Create a raster algebra expression for the index

The next set of steps is tedious, but the model has the advantage of storing the steps and expression for correction or revision, if necessary. Note: If you are unsuccessful in creating the needed Raster Calculator expression, you can copy and paste it from the bottom of the Statistics.txt file.

1 **In ArcToolbox, with Spatial Analyst Tools expanded, expand the Map Algebra toolset, drag the Single Output Map Algebra tool to the right side of your model and drop it there.**

Do not open it yet.

2 **From the Spatial Analyst menu, click Raster Calculator.**

While you want the expression for the Map Algebra tool, it's easier to create it in the Raster Calculator and then paste into the tool's form.

3 **Create the expression as follows, using keypad buttons as much as possible and copying and pasting statistics from Statistics.txt.**

Be careful to put spaces on both sides of operators such as "-", "+", and "/" (the keypad buttons in the Raster Calculator will do this for you automatically). Spaces are not needed for parentheses or raster layer names. *Do not click the Evaluate button yet!*

$$(((([male16unem] - 3.439298600438196e\text{-}005) / 3.061485872188322e\text{-}005) + (([poverty] - 3.8945716740923e\text{-}005) / 3.731077384784302e\text{-}005) + (([nohighsch] - 2.523184009633747e\text{-}005) / 1.794571104479892e\text{-}005) + (([fhhchld] - 7.88028756106625e\text{-}006) / 1.06967128765136e\text{-}005)) / 4$$

4   Select your finished expression from the Raster Calculator, press Ctrl+C to copy the expression.

5   Click Evaluate.

If your result is correct, a new Calculation layer will be added to ArcMap, showing values of -1.07748 to 3.96905. If not, repeat steps 2 and 3, looking closely for errors or omissions. If you are unsuccessful, use the expression at the bottom of Statistics.txt.

6   Right-click the Single Output Map Algebra tool in your model and click Open.

7   Click inside the Map Algebra expression panel and press Ctrl+V to paste your expression from the Raster Calculator.

8   Set the Output raster path to **\GistutorialHealth\SpatialAnalyst\PovertyIndex**, expand the Input raster or feature data option, and add the four input layers shown in the graphic below.

The latter part just causes the model to show arrow lines between the inputs and the Single Output Map Algebra tool element.

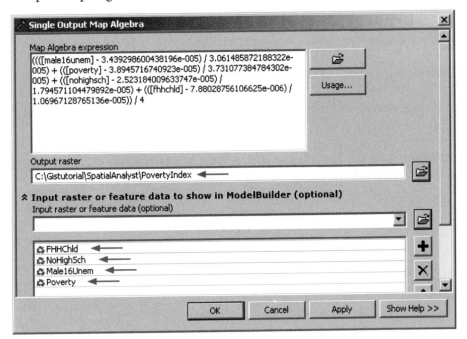

9   Click OK and click the AutoLayout button in ModelBuilder. ∎

Run the model

All but the last model element have already been run, so you will run it now.

1 Right-click Single Output Map Algebra and rename it **Create Poverty Index Raster.**

2 Right-click PovertyIndex and click Add to Display.

3 Save your model.

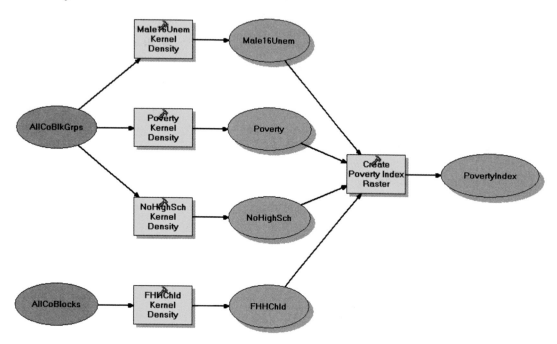

4 Right-click Create Poverty Index Raster, click Run, and then Close.

5 Add the Poverty Index to your display and close the model.

Note: If you wish to change or run your model after you close it, right-click it in ArcToolbox and click Edit.

6 Resymbolize the new layer using the Classified method, a Standard Deviation classification with 1/3 Std Dev interval size, and the green-yellow-red color ramp.

Create poverty contour

Suppose that after trial and error, policy analysts wish to use the poverty index of 1.0 or higher to define poverty. Next, you will create a shapefile that has the contour line for that index "elevation."

1   In ArcToolbox, with the Spatial Analyst Tools expanded, expand the Surface toolset, and double-click the Contour List tool.

2   Type or make the selections shown below.

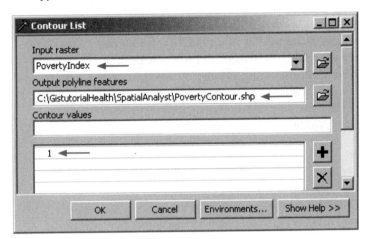

3   Click OK.

You now have a set of polygons that explicitly define poverty areas and can be used for many additional purposes.

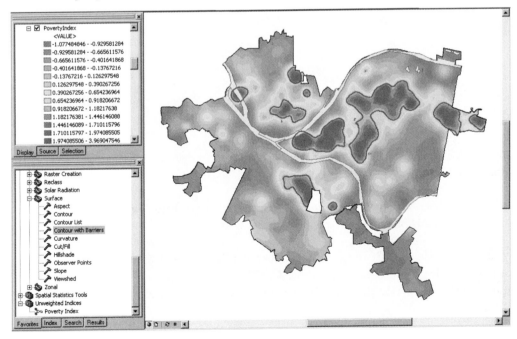

4   Save the map document and close ArcMap.

Summary

This study has produced many valuable outputs in support of locating defibrillators in public places in Pittsburgh. You discovered that only a few areas are large enough in demand to meet the criterion of having commercial land uses. You can also explain that heart attack incidence rates and population determine only a part of the spatial distribution of heart attacks that occur in public places. Finally, you have constructed a useful index and contour lines defining poverty in Pittsburgh, which are useful in explaining heart attacks and for many other purposes.

On the technical side, you have become quite sophisticated users of raster GIS and ArcGIS Spatial Analyst. You can work with and enhance raster maps, such as for elevation and land use, using masks to display irregularly shaped study areas and hillshade to give a three-dimensional appearance that is attractive. You have a working knowledge of density maps and how to create them using kernel density smoothing in ArcGIS Spatial Analyst. You know how to query raster maps. Finally, you can process raster maps, combining them with map algebra, and build impressive macros via ModelBuilder.

References

Dawes, R. M. 1979. The robust beauty of improper linear models in decision making. *American Psychologist* 34: 571–82.

The Harvard Medical School Family Health Guide. Public defibrillators. http://www.health.harvard. edu/fhg/updates/update0504a.shtml. Accessed July 26, 2008.

O'Hare, W., and M. Mather. 2003. The growing number of kids in severely distressed neighborhoods: Evidence from the 2000 census. *Kids Count*, a publication of the Annie E. Casey Foundation and the Population Reference Bureau. http://www.aefc.org/upload/publicationfiles /da3622h1280.pdf.

Rosamond, W. D., L. E. Chambless, A. R. Folsom, L. S. Cooper, D. E. Conwill, L. Clegg, C. H. Wang, and G. Heiss. 1998. Trends in incidence of myocardial infarction and in mortality due to coronary heart disease, 1987 to 1994. *New England Journal of Medicine* 339: 861–67.

Exercise assignment 9-1

Display schools and land use for locating school-based health centers

Problem:

The first ring of suburbs around urban areas may undergo revitalization in the future as suburban homeowners attempt to downsize houses and relocate closer to work. In anticipation of this growth in Pittsburgh, suppose that the Allegheny County Health Department plans to create satellite centers located in these suburbs' schools. The centers will provide flu shots, health wellness education programs, lead poisoning prevention programs, and other services. As a starting point for choosing potential schools for these centers, this assignment has you prepare a map with land use and school locations for the first ring of suburbs.

You will choose the appropriate subset of municipalities in Allegheny County, create a mask for them, and use the mask to display land use with hillshade. Then you will add a layers for schools and display those in the same area.

Start with the following:

- **C:\GistutorialHealth\SpatialAnalyst\Munic.shp**—polygon layer for municipalities in Allegheny County.

- **C:\GistutorialHealth\SpatialAnalyst\CountySchools.dbf**—XY data file that has names of schools and (x,y) point coordinates in Pennsylvania south state plane 1983 projection.

- **C:\GistutorialHealth\SpatialArclyst\Pittsburgh.shp**—Boundary polygon for Pittsburgh.

- **C:\GistutorialHealth\SpatialAnalyst\LandUse\28910720.tif**—land use for Allegheny County.

- **C:\GistutorialHealth\SpatialAnalyst\DEM**—digital elevation model for Allegheny County.

- **C:\GistutorialHealth\SpatialAnalyst\LandUsePgh.lyr**—layer file for rendering land-use raster.

Preprocess vector layers

In ArcMap, create a map document called C:\GistutorialHealth\Answers\Assignment9\Assignment9-1.mxd with each of the above layers added. *Add the municipalities first,* so that your data frame inherits that layer's projection, which is the local 1983 state plane projection. When creating a hillshade, you'll rely on the data frame having state frame coordinates (in feet) so that the hillshade gets the same coordinates. Use Tools, Add XY Data for county schools. Reset the source for LandUsePgh.lyr to \GistutorialHealth\SpatialAnalyst \LandUse\28910720.tif by opening its property sheet. Turn off Pittsburgh.shp to simplify the next step, where you'll create a ring of suburbs.

Define the first ring of suburbs as those within one mile of Pittsburgh, but not including Pittsburgh in Munic.shp. Start by clicking Selection, Set Selectable Layers, and make Munic the only selectable layer for now. Then use Selection, Select by Location, and select municipalities that are within a distance of one mile of Pittsburgh. Then use the Select Features tool, hold down your Shift key, and click inside the Pittsburgh polygon in the Munic.shp layer to deselect it. (Hint: To verify you are deselecting Pittsburgh, see the number of selected features reported at the bottom left of the ArcMap window.) That leaves the ring of suburbs selected, with a hole in the center. Finally, right-click Munic, and click Data, Export data to create \Assignment9\suburbs.shp and add it to your map document. Now select schools that intersect with suburbs.shp and create \Assignment9\suburbanschools.shp.

Set environment and create mask

Set ArcToolbox's environment: Under General Settings, make the \Assignment9 folder the current workspace, make the Output Coordinate System be the Same as Layer "Munic" (this is critically important, so that your raster layer gets state plane coordinates in feet), and use suburbs.shp as the extent. Under Raster Analysis Settings, set a 50-foot cell size. Convert suburbs.shp into a raster layer (cell size 50) called \Assignment9\submask. Now reset the environment so that the mask and extent point to submask.

Process raster layers

Using the new mask, extract a raster from 28910720.tif (\Assignment9\SubLandUse), and import the land-use layer file for symbolization. Set the options for the Spatial Analyst toolbar to *use the active frame's coordinate system for output,* SubLandUse for the mask and extent, with a cell size of 50, then create a hillshade from DEM (\Assignment9\Hillshade). Symbolize Hillshade so that it has sufficient contrast. (Make sublanduse semi-transparent, move it above the hillshade, turn off unneeded layers, and turn on the suburban schools to display them with the hillshade and sublanduse layers). Housing will be in the red, developed areas. Export your map to C:\GistutorialHealth\Answers\Assignment9\Assignment9-1.pdf.

Exercise assignment 9-2

Determine heart attack fatalities outside of hospitals in Mount Lebanon by gender

Unfortunately, females have more fatal heart attacks outside of hospitals than males, perhaps because symptoms of heart attacks in females are less well known than those for males. Heart attacks outside of hospitals are roughly 1.5 per thousand for males aged 35 to 74 and 2.3 for females in the same age range. In this assignment, you will create two density map layers using these incidence rates for the municipality of Mount Lebanon in Allegheny County, one for males and one for females. You will do all raster processing using Spatial Analysis tools in a model.

Start with the following:

- **C:\GistutorialHealth\SpatialAnalyst\Munic.shp**—polygon layer for municipalities in Allegheny County.

- **C:\GistutorialHealth\SpatialAnalyst\AllCoBlocks.shp**—point layer for census block centroids in Allegheny County.

In ArcMap, create a map document called C:\GistutorialHealth\Answers\Assignment9\Assignment9-2.mxd with the above layers added. Select the Mount Lebanon polygon from munic.shp and export it as C:\GistutorialHealth \Answers\Assignment9\MtLebanon.shp. Add floating point fields to the attribute table for AllCoBlocks.shp: MMortinc = [Male35T74] × 0.0015 for the annual number of heart attack fatalities for males aged 35 to 74 and FMortinc = [Fem35T74] × 0.0023 for females aged 35 to 74.

Create a new toolbox called Disease Incidence, stored in the \Assignment9 folder. Create a model in the new toolbox called HeartAttack.

Working in your model, use MtLebanon.shp to create a raster layer called \Assignment9\MtLebanon.img with the extent of MtLebanon.shp and cell size 30. Create kernel density map layers for MMortinc and FMortinc using MtLebanon.img as the mask with a cell size of 100 and search radius of 1,500 square feet. (Hint: Use the Kernel Density tool in ArcToolbox.) Give the outputs descriptive names, add them to the map in two separate data frames, apply the same symbology scheme to both, and create a layout comparing male and female out-of-hospital heart-attack fatalities in Mt. Lebanon, Pennsylvania, from 2000 to 2005. Export your map as C:\GistutorialHealth\Answers\Assignment9\Assignments9-2.pdf.

What to turn in

If you are working in a classroom setting with an instructor, you may be required to submit the files that you created for chapter 9. Below are files that you are required to turn in. Be sure to use a compression program such as PKZIP or WinZip to include all files as one ZIP document for review and grading. Include your name and assignment number in the ZIP document <YourNameAssignment9.zip>.

ArcMap files

C:\GistutorialHealth\Answers\Assignment9\Assignment9-1.mxd
C:\GistutorialHealth\Answers\Assignment9\Assignment9-2.mxd

Toolbox

C:\GistutorialHealth\Answers\Assignment9\Disease_Incidence.tbx

Shapefiles

C:\GistutorialHealth\Answers\Assignment9\suburbs.shp
C:\GistutorialHealth\Answers\Assignment9\suburbanschools.shp
C:\GistutorialHealth\Answers\Assignment9\MtLebanon.shp

Rasters

C:\GistutorialHealth\Answers\Assignment9\submask
C:\GistutorialHealth\Answers\Assignment9\Hillshade
C:\GistutorialHealth\Answers\Assignment9\SubLandUse
C:\GistutorialHealth\Answers\Assignment9\MtLebanon.img
(Be sure to include all files associated with the rasters.)

Exported maps

C:\GistutorialHealth\Answers\Assignment9\Assignment9-1.pdf
C:\GistutorialHealth\Answers\Assignment9\Assignment9-2.pdf

OBJECTIVES

Assemble basemaps for emergency preparedness
Geocode events to trace an outbreak source
Use buffer analysis to identify affected office buildings
Use buffer analysis to access vulnerable populations

GIS Tutorial 10

Case study: Studying food-borne disease outbreaks

Introduction

You likely will want to use GIS in projects for your own organization, research, or other purposes. Such work requires that you clarify the problem or issue to be studied, identify a solution that employs GIS, determine what data and other resources are available, then design a workflow that progresses from intermediate answers to final presentations for clients and other audiences. You will use many project management and applied research skills for such work, beyond merely understanding the functionality available in ArcGIS.

Tutorials 1 through 9 have helped you build your knowledge of both available GIS functionality and workflows through parts or phases of GIS projects. This tutorial and the final tutorial will have you working on case studies, doing independent GIS project work. You will learn no new GIS functionality; rather, you will learn how to structure project work and carry out longer sequences of steps that integrate across the previous tutorials. Tutorials 10 and 11 each have a health scenario as before, but do not provide step-by-step instructions. Instead, we provide guidelines for carrying out GIS project work and have you follow them while deciding on the particular steps to take.

Health-care scenario

According to the Centers of Disease Control and Prevention (CDC), food can transmit more than 200 known diseases caused by bacteria and viruses. The CDC estimates approximately 76 million cases of food-borne illnesses occur in the United States each year, accounting for 325,000 hospitalizations and 5,000 deaths (Meade, et al. 1999). In addition to such naturally occurring threats, health organizations—including state and local health departments—are concerned about food-borne illness in connection to emergency preparedness and homeland security. For example, in grocery stores and restaurants, terrorists could taint food with infectious agents.

GIS can be used to track and analyze disease outbreaks caused by food-borne agents, including the exposure of populations to risks and the availability of surrounding health services. With GIS, you could quickly map reported illnesses from food contaminations and model populations at risk for other outbreaks.

In this case study, you will prepare maps to analyze scenarios of food-borne disease outbreaks in Allegheny County, Pennsylvania. Members of the Allegheny County Health Department's Food Safety Program inspect and regulate every type of food establishment and investigate food contamination and food-borne illnesses.

Case-study requirements

The major deliverable for the case study is a computer folder with shapefiles, map documents, a Microsoft PowerPoint presentation, and a project report suitable for the director of the health department.

The following is an outline and guidelines for the project report. Use each category listed below in the order given as sections in your report. In addition to the report, create a PowerPoint presentation with bullets for major parts of each section in your report. The PowerPoint presentation should also include output maps and tables.

Problem definition and solution approach

Write a short introduction that includes the definition of the problem, the solution approach, and the scope of the project, including limitations.

- *Clearly state the problem, opportunity, issue, or objective.* The problem is often a gap between the current and desired state of a region—for example, too many uninsured persons in a state or too few safe play areas in poor parts of a city.
- *Provide an approach for the solution.* The approach identifies performance measures for the phenomenon under investigation. For example, the number or percent of uninsured adults by county may be a performance measure if programs exist or could exist to reduce it, and the percentage of children living within five minutes of a park may be a performance measure if there are or could be housing programs designed to increase this number. The approach also identifies major data sources and, therefore, the feasibility of the project.
- *Define the scope or limitations of the project.* Most projects do not have the resources and data that would be needed to accomplish all that can be envisioned as desirable. Thus, it is important to state the scope and any limitations. For example, scope might include studying the number of uninsured, but not the availability of other options for health care, such as low-cost clinics. A limitation may be that because of the unavailability of data, the study includes only county-level data on the uninsured, even though census-tract-level data would be helpful.

Data

Describe the data you will use for your project—its sources, descriptions, and locations within the project's computer file folders.

- *Describe the inputs to your project and their sources.* Search for "Internet citations" on the Internet and pick a style for referencing Web sources. Use that style to provide citations for download sites and other data sources.
- *Create a computer folder, subfolders, and file structure for the project.* At a minimum, create a project folder and subfolders for data tables (for attribute data), map layers, and documents.

Methodology

Write a high-level description of methodologies used. For example, you can say that you used ArcGIS and Microsoft Excel software to create the GIS data and produce results, you placed injury data on the map through geocoding, and you then did a proximity analysis using buffers.

- *Create an outline of steps for data preparation.* These steps, and the steps under the next two bullets, should be detailed enough so that a GIS user could carry them out. Examples are (1) delete all columns except identifiers, elderly population (age 65 and older), and poverty measures from the SF3 census data table; (2) create new columns for percent of elderly population that lives in poverty.

- *Create an outline of steps for constructing GIS data.* Examples are (1) geocode an injury table using a TIGER/Line street map layer to produce the Injuries point layer; (2) classify the injury point layer by neighborhood using the neighborhood polygon layer and a spatial join, and so forth.
- *Create an outline of steps for spatial analysis.* Examples are (1) create 500-, 1,000-, and 5,000-foot buffers for the parks layer; (2) use spatial joins of the buffers and injuries point layer, and so on.

Results

This section presents and discusses output maps and tables and also summarizes the results or findings of the case study. Point out interesting patterns and limitations to the reader and refer to each exhibit by number. Place each map and table on the page following its first mention in the text. In a Microsoft Word document and PowerPoint presentation you will do the following:

- *Prepare professional-quality map layouts and statistical tables with results.*
- *Write short descriptions of the results, referring to figure and table numbers.*

Discussion and future work

In this section, you interpret your results and make the recommendations and suggestions for future work that will remove limitations or expand the scope of analysis.

Part 1: Assemble basemaps

Scenario:

During an emergency, analysts need to have data readily available so they can respond quickly with appropriate actions. A real-time monitoring system, with a complete and comprehensive set of GIS base layers, needs to be in place and ready for interactive use by a GIS analyst.

In this section, you will use the following layers to create a GIS basemap that could be used to analyze food-borne disease outbreaks. You will use street centerlines for the city of Pittsburgh and geocode food sources by street location. This will allow the health department to quickly identify possible sources for food-borne contaminations. Copy all tables and layers to your project folders.

Start with the following:

- **C:\GistutorialHealth\PAGIS\Neighborhood.shp**—polygon shapefile of neighborhood outlines.

- **C:\GistutorialHealth\PAGIS\StreetsCL.shp**—line shapefile of street centerlines.

- **C:\GistutorialHealth\PAGIS\Sidewalks.shp**—line shapefile of sidewalks.

- **C:\GistutorialHealth\PAGIS\Buildings.shp**—polygon shapefile of Pittsburgh building outlines.

- **C:\GistutorialHealth\ACHD\PghFoodSources.dbf**—a table of food sources from the Allegheny County Health Department.

Note: The data is from food inspections but has been modified for privacy protection. After geocoding, create separate layers for the following four food establishment types as determined by the supplied query conditions. This will help epidemiologist and emergency planners quickly analyze which types of establishments might be a potential cause for a food-borne outbreak.

The following describes the various food sources in the PghFoodSources database:

Bakeries	Bakery or Chain Bakery
Restaurants	Adult Food Service Adult Food Service Fee Exempt Chain Restaurant with Liquor Chain Restaurant without Liquor Restaurant without Liquor Restaurant with Liquor
Grocery stores	Supermarket Chain Supermarket
Convenience stores	Chain Retail Convenience Store

To do:

1   Create a GIS project with the above layers and food sources geocoded to Pittsburgh streets.

2   Rematch as many food locations as possible.

3   Create a map layout of buildings, streets, sidewalks, neighborhoods, and food sources by type.

4   In a Word document, keep a log of the steps you took to rematch your addresses. What are some reasons that the food sources did not match? Describe what additional steps may be needed for all food sources to match. Include the log as an appendix in your report.

Part 2: Trace an outbreak source

Scenario:

City hospitals report unusually high numbers of the food-borne illness hepatitis A. Home addresses of patients who are affected and their work addresses are available as data. Because you already have a basemap for analysis, you can quickly create a map that shows the residences and work locations of the affected patients to determine possible outbreak locations.

Other information that you know about the patients includes the following:

• None ate at restaurants that serve alcohol.

• Most patients were very busy and had quick lunches within two or three blocks of where they worked (about a 500-foot buffer).

Start with the following:

• Map document from part 1 of this case study.

• **C:\GistutorialHealth\ACHD\OutbreakResidences.dbf.**

• **C:\GistutorialHealth\ACHD\OutbreakWorkLocations.dbf.**

To do:

1 Geocode outbreak residences and work locations, and add the results to the map composition of part 1. What observations do you make from the finished map?

2 Using the information from above, determine what restaurants are possible sources for the outbreak.

3 In your report, name the restaurants that are possible risks.

4 Create a map layout showing the results of your analysis.

Part 3: Identify affected office buildings

Scenario:

Given a known infectious source, it is useful for public health officials to determine the buildings in which likely patrons of an establishment would work or live. Then those individuals could be informed of the known infection/violation and advised to seek immediate help if they start displaying certain symptoms. In the case of a contagious outbreak of a pathogen from a point source, a similar process could be used to identify buildings for quarantine or evacuation. Again, a walking distance measure would identify buildings containing at-risk or potentially infected individuals.

In this scenario, food safety officials determined that the fictional restaurant called "Generic Deli" was found to be the source of the food contamination.

Start with the following:

- Map documents and layers from parts 1 and 2 of this case study.

To do:

1 Create a map with a layer of buildings within the Pittsburgh neighborhood where patients work, a quarter-mile buffer around Generic Deli, and buildings whose centers are completely within this buffer.

2 Create a map layout showing the results of your analysis and a description of how you approached the problem.

Part 4: Assess vulnerable populations

Scenario:

Public health officials need to estimate the areas and populations at risk from an identified infectious source, namely, where potential customers of an identified source reside, how many particularly susceptible individuals (in this case, population 5 and under, and 65 and over) might be affected, and what the maximum number of potential cases is. This information would be useful for response planning, including communication, identification of new cases, and ensuring sufficient treatment facilities, supplies of antibiotics, and available personnel.

In this scenario, Pittsburgh's rivers flooded. After the flood waters receded, food establishments within flood zones reopened. Due to power outages in these areas, the health department needs to inspect these establishments to make sure they have properly disposed of affected food supplies and cleaned food preparation areas and equipment. The health department wants to know the elderly (65 and over) and very young (5 and under) populations within half-mile and one-mile buffers of these food sources so that they can prioritize their inspections.

Start with the following:

- Geocoded food sources from part 1.

- **C:\GistutorialHealth\PAGIS\BlockCentroids.shp**—point shapefile of census blocks that includes Summary File 1 (SF1) data.

- **C:\GistutorialHealth\PAGIS\FemaFlood.shp**—polygon shapefile of flood zones.

To do:

1   Create maps showing the food establishments within the flood zones, polygon buffers of a half-mile and one mile around these establishments, census block centroids, a count of total population within each buffer, census block centroids showing population 65 and over only, and a count of population 65 and over within each buffer; and census block centroids showing a population 5 and under only, and a count of total population 5 and under within each buffer.

2   Create a map layout and a table showing the results of your analysis.

What to turn in:

If you are working in a classroom setting with an instructor, you may be required to submit the exercises you created in chapter 10. Below are the files you are required to turn in. Be sure to use a compression program such as PKZIP or WinZip to include all files as one ZIP document for review and grading. Include your name and assignment number in the ZIP document <YourNameCaseStudy1.zip>.

Folders containing map documents, shapefiles, data tables, images, and so on.

C:\GistutorialHealth\Answers\Casestudy1\YourFolders

Final report—Word document

C:\GistutorialHealth\Answers\Casestudy1\FinalReport.doc

Final presentation—PowerPoint document

C:\GistutorialHealth\Answers\Casestudy1\FinalPresentation.ppt

Reference

Mead, P. S., L. Slutsker, D. Vance, L. F. McCaig, J. S. Bresee, C. Shapiro, P. M. Griffin, and R. V. Tauxe. 1999. Food-related illness and death in the United States. *Emerging infectious diseases* 5, no. 5, 607.

OBJECTIVES

Perform market analysis
Perform territory analysis
Track chapter status

GIS Tutorial 11

Case study: Forming a national ACHE chapter

Here, as in tutorial 11, you will work on a case study independently. We give you a health scenario as before, but do not provide step-by-step instructions. Instead, we provide guidelines for carrying out GIS project work and ask you to follow them while making your own decisions on the particular steps to take.

Health-care scenario

The American College of Healthcare Executives (ACHE) based in Chicago, Illinois, is the leading professional association of health-care executives worldwide. ACHE has a 70-year history of serving executives across the health-care industry by providing new educational opportunities, media products and services, professional credentialing, career development services, and networking opportunities.

To respond to the changing needs of the health-care management profession, ACHE developed a plan to form a network of local independent chapters that would be closer to where members lived and still provide the standard ACHE programs and benefits.

Recently, the ACHE board of governors formalized its plans to evaluate and develop chapters by starting its "Partners for Success" chapter deployment project. The final chapter network consists of independent, separate corporations bound by an agreement with ACHE. Existing affiliate groups—Healthcare Executive Groups and Women Health Executive Networks (HEG_WHEN)—formed initial ACHE chapters and new chapters are being developed to fill gaps in coverage.

One of the major steps of the project is to determine where health-care executive chapters should be located to create better regional coverage. In this case study, you will create maps for this purpose. You will use the maps to determine if the desired market areas are unique, nonoverlapping, and cover areas with demand. In the case-study scenario, you will have the role of GIS analyst working for ACHE.

We expect that there will be many opportunities in the future to draw on networks of organizations for providing health care and that designing territories for responsibilities will be an integral part of such work. Analysts will need to carry out similar studies in a competitive environment as well, mapping their own territories and those of others.

Case-study requirements

As in the previous case study in tutorial 10, the major deliverable for the case study is a computer folder containing shapefiles, map documents, a Microsoft PowerPoint presentation, and a project report suitable for the board of governors for the American College of Healthcare Executives.

Follow the case-study requirements already described in tutorial 10 for problem definition and solution approach, data, methodology, results, and discussion and future work.

Phase 1: Creating market analysis maps

In phase 1, you will perform a market analysis based on ACHE membership data by ZIP Code obtained from its affiliate groups. You will conduct a proximity analysis using 25-, 50-, 75-, and 100-mile concentric buffers of affiliate office locations with members by ZIP Code. The resulting maps will allow ACHE chapter leaders to identify overlapping territories. GIS-generated maps could then be made available to leaders of potential new chapters, who could survey uncovered areas for selecting counties and ZIP Codes of new territories.

The figure below is a diagram similar to one you can build to automate the steps to create maps for a market analysis.

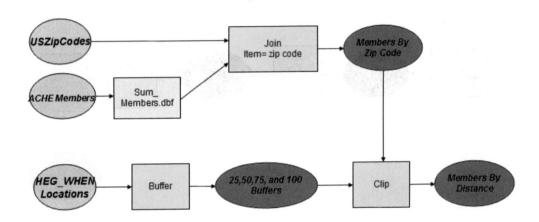

American College of Healthcare Executives
Market Analysis

Start with the following:

- **C:\GistutorialHealth\UnitedStates\States.shp**—polygon shapefile of U.S. states with current ACHE districts (field=DISTRICT).

- **C:\GistutorialHealth\ACHE\ACHEMembers.dbf**—table of current ACHE members by ZIP Code. Hint: summarize the ACHEMembers.dbf file on the ZIP field, then join this file to ZIP Code polygons.

- **C:\GistutorialHealth\ACHE\HEG_WHEN.shp**—point shapefile of existing Healthcare Executive Groups and Women Health Executive Networks.

- **C:\GistutorialHealth\UnitedStates\ZipCodes.shp**—polygon shapefile of ZIP Codes for the United States.

Create a series of maps that include current ACHE districts, a choropleth map of ACHE members per ZIP Code, and multiple buffers of 25, 50, 75, and 100 miles of HEG_WHEN locations.

Phase 2: Creating a territory analysis map

The ACHE Partners for Success prospectus contains 18 criteria and a number of tools to help leaders of prospective new chapters evaluate their readiness to become an ACHE chapter. Several of the criteria address territory analysis.

During phase 2 mapping, you will identify overlapping areas. Potential chapter leaders can then make decisions to add or drop ZIP Codes or counties from their proposed service areas to eliminate overlaps. The same maps can also be used in negotiations between various adjoining chapters.

The figure below is similar to one that you can build to automate the steps to create maps for a territory analysis.

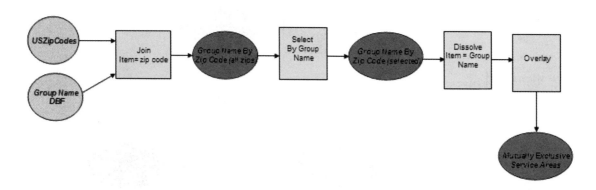

Start with the following:

- **C:\GistutorialHealth\ACHE\GroupsDistricts1_2_3.dbf**—table of ACHE group partners by ZIP Code for districts 1–3.

- **C:\GistutorialHealth\ACHE\GroupsDistricts4_5_6.dbf**—table of ACHE group partners by ZIP Code for districts 4–6.

- **C:\GistutorialHealth\ACHE\ZipCodes.shp**—polygon shapefile of ZIP Codes for the United States.

- **C:\GistutorialHealth\UnitedStates\States.shp**—polygon shapefile of U.S. states.

- **ACHE_Districts.shp**—polygon shapefile created in phase 1 marketing of the case study.

Create maps showing territories for overlapping affiliate groups in districts 1, 2, and 3.

The group districts database includes affiliate groups with overlapping ZIP Codes. In order to see the overlap, you need to extract each group to its own database, join the new database of each group to U.S. ZIP Code features, extract just ZIP Codes for each group, and dissolve on the group name. Your table of contents should include a separate layer/shapefile for each dissolved group territory.

Build a model for the above process and include a screen capture of the model in your final presentation and report. Hint: If you have trouble repeating the model, remove existing joins on the ZIP Code features before rerunning the model.

Show each group territory as transparent polygons or hollow outlines to see the groups that overlap.

Create a new shapefile of overlapping group territories in New York, Pennsylvania, and Ohio. Show the overlapping areas with a crosshatch fill.

For extra practice, repeat the above steps for groups in districts 4, 5, and 6.

These maps will give affiliate group planners and leaders and ACHE staff their first determination of which territories overlap. Affiliate groups with overlapping territories are required to contact each other to coordinate boundaries or consider a merger/alliance. When finished, a new file containing counties and ZIP Codes making up the realigned territory will be sent to ACHE for remapping.

During conference calls, territory maps can be reviewed and counties and ZIP Codes can be added or deleted from a territory.

Phase 3: Tracking chapter status

After potential chapters submit their proposals for being chartered with ACHE, they are either given Chartered Chapter Status or, if not all provisions are accepted, they are given Provisional Chapter Status.

Chicago ACHE staff use the Chapter Status Tracking System to keep track of an applicant's progress in meeting criteria. The system also tracks unclaimed territory—whole or partial counties not claimed by a chapter.

Start with the following:

- **C:\GistutorialHealth\ACHE\ResolvedPartners.dbf**—table of ACHE resolved group partners by ZIP Code.

  The Partners.dbf file contains an item "Status" with values:
  - PCHP = Provisional (able to meet 11 of the 18 criteria for chartered status)
  - CHP = Chartered (all 18 criteria for becoming an ACHE Chapter Corporation are met)

- **C:\GistutorialHealth\ACHE\ZipCodes.shp**—polygon shapefile of ZIP Codes for the United States.

Create maps showing which chapters are provisional and which are chartered for each ACHE district. Export your maps as JPEG images and add them to your final presentation document.

What to turn in:

If you are working in a classroom setting with an instructor, you may be required to submit the exercises you created in chapter 11. Below are the files you are required to turn in. Be sure to use a compression program such as PKZIP or WinZip to include all files as one ZIP document for review and grading. Include your name and assignment number in the ZIP document <YourNameCaseStudy2.zip>

Folders containing map documents, shapefiles, data tables, images, and so forth
C:\GistutorialHealth\Answers\Casestudy2\YourFolders

Final report—Word document
C:\GistutorialHealth\Answers\Casestudy2\FinalReport.doc

Final presentation—PowerPoint document
C:\GistutorialHealth\Answers\Casestudy2\FinalPresentation.ppt

Appendix A

Data source credits

Tutorial 1 figure sources include:

Figure 1.1- Lung cancer mortality per 100,000 white males, 1970-1994

\GistutorialHealth\UnitedStates\MajorCities.shp, from ESRI Data & Maps 2004, courtesy of U.S. Census.

\GistutorialHealth\UnitedStates\Rivers.shp, from ESRI Data & Maps 2004, courtesy of ArcWorld.

\GistutorialHealth\UnitedStates\Interstates.shp, from ESRI Data & Maps 2004, courtesy of U.S. Bureau of Transportation Statistics.

\GistutorialHealth\UnitedStates\Lakes.shp, from ESRI Data & Maps 2004, courtesy of ArcWorld.

\GistutorialHealth\UnitedStates\States.shp, from ESRI Data & Maps 2007, courtesy of ArcUSA, U.S. Census, ESRI (Pop2005 field).

\GistutorialHealth\UnitedStates\Counties.shp, from ESRI Data & Maps 2007, courtesy of ArcUSA, U.S. Census, ESRI (Pop2005 field).

\GistutorialHealth\LungCounty_7094.shp, created by joining Counties.shp with lungcounty.xls from The Cancer Mortality Maps & Graphs Web Site, courtesy of the National Cancer Society.

Figure 1.2- Locations of serious injuries to child pedestrians in Eastern Pittsburgh, Pennsylvania

\GistutorialHealth\PedestrianInjuries\InjuriesJones.shp, courtesy of Children's Hospital of Pittsburgh and U.S. Census Bureau TIGER.

\GistutorialHealth\PAGIS\pittsburgh_east_pa_ne.tif, courtesy of Pennsylvania Spatial Data Access (PASDA) and USGS.

\GistutorialHealth\PAGIS\ParksPlaygrounds.shp, courtesy of the City of Pittsburgh, Department of City Planning.

Tutorial 1 data sources include:

\GistutorialHealth\UnitedStates\States.shp, from ESRI Data & Maps, 2007, courtesy of ArcUSA, U.S. Census, ESRI (Pop2005 field).

\GistutorialHealth\UnitedStates\MajorCities.shp, from ESRI Data & Maps 2004 courtesy of U.S. Census.

\GistutorialHealth\UnitedStates\Rivers.shp, from ESRI Data & Maps 2004, courtesy of ArcWorld.

\GistutorialHealth\UnitedStates\Lakes.shp, from ESRI Data & Maps 2004, courtesy of ArcWorld.

\GistutorialHealth\UnitedStates\Interstates.shp, from ESRI Data & Maps 2004, courtesy of U.S. Bureau of Transportation Statistics.

\GistutorialHealth\UnitedStates\Counties.shp, from ESRI Data & Maps 2007, courtesy of ArcUSA, U.S. Census, ESRI (Pop2005 field).

\GistutorialHealth\NCI\LungCounty_7094.shp, created by joining Counties.shp with lungcounty.xls from The Cancer Mortality Maps & Graphs Web Site, courtesy of the National Cancer Society.

Tutorial 2 data sources include:

\GistutorialHealth\UnitedStates\States.shp, from ESRI Data & Maps, 2007, courtesy of ArcUSA, U.S. Census, ESRI (Pop2005 field).

\GistutorialHealth\UnitedStates\MajorCities.shp, from ESRI Data & Maps 2004, courtesy of U.S. Census.

\GistutorialHealth\NCI\BreState5_9094.shp, from The Cancer Mortality Maps & Graphs Web Site, courtesy of The National Cancer Institute.

\GistutorialHealth\NCI\BreCounty_7094.shp, from The Cancer Mortality Maps & Graphs Web Site, courtesy of The National Cancer Institute.

\GistutorialHealth\UnitedStates\Counties.shp, from ESRI Data & Maps 2007, courtesy of ArcUSA, U.S. Census, ESRI (Pop2005 field).

\GistutorialHealth\NCI\LungState5_9094.shp, from The Cancer Mortality Maps & Graphs Web Site, courtesy of The National Cancer Institute.

\GistutorialHealth\NCI\LungCounty_7094.shp, from The Cancer Mortality Maps & Graphs Web Site, courtesy of The National Cancer Institute.

Tutorial 3 data sources include:

\GistutorialHealth\Texas\Counties.shp, from ESRI Data & Maps 2007, courtesy of ArcUSA, U.S. Census, ESRI (Pop2005 field).

\GistutorialHealth\California\Counties.shp, from ESRI Data & Maps 2007, courtesy of ArcUSA, U.S. Census, ESRI (Pop2005 field).

\GistutorialHealth\Texas\HarrisCensusTracts.shp,,courtesy of U.S. Census Bureau TIGER.

\GistutorialHealth\Texas\HarrisCountyCities.shp, from ESRI Data & Maps 2004, courtesy of National Atlas of the United States.

Tutorial 4 data sources include:

\GistutorialHealth\World\World_30.shp, from ESRI Data & Maps 2002, courtesy of ESRI.

\GistutorialHealth\World\AIDSCases.shp, from ESRI Data & Maps 2005, courtesy of ESRI and U.S. Census.

\GistutorialHealth\UnitedStates\States.shp, from ESRI Data & Maps 2007, courtesy of ArcUSA, U.S. Census, ESRI (Popfield 2005).

\GistutorialHealth\UnitedStates\Lakes.shp, from ESRI Data & Maps 2004, courtesy of ArcWorld.

\GistutorialHealth\NCI\LungCounty_7094.shp, created by joining Counties.shp with lungcounty.xls from The Cancer Mortality Maps & Graphs Web Site, courtesy of the National Cancer Society.

\GistutorialHealth\PAGIS\NeighStatePlane.shp, courtesy of the City of Pittsburgh, Department of City Planning.

\GistutorialHealth\PAGIS\Neighborhoods.shp, courtesy of the City of Pittsburgh, Department of City Planning.

\GistutorialHealth\PAGIS\Sidewalks.shp, courtesy of the City of Pittsburgh, Department of City Planning.

\GistutorialHealth\PAGIS\Parks.shp, courtesy of the City of Pittsburgh, Department of City Planning.

\GistutorialHealth\PAGIS\Rivers.shp, courtesy of the City of Pittsburgh, Department of City Planning.

\GistutorialHealth\PAGIS\Topo25ft.shp, courtesy of the City of Pittsburgh, Department of City Planning.

\GistutorialHealth\Pennsylvania\tr42_d00.e00, courtesy of U.S. Census Bureau TIGER.

\GistutorialHealth\Pennsylvania\PASchools.dbf, from ESRI Data & Maps, 2005, courtesy of USGS.

\GistutorialHealth\PAGIS\pittsburgh_east_pa_ne.tif, courtesy of Pennsylvania Spatial Data Access (PASDA) and USGS.

\GistutorialHealth\World\InfantMortalityRates.shp, from ESRI Data & Maps, 2005, courtesy of ESRI and U.S. Census.

\GistutorialHealth\PAGIS\Buildings.shp, courtesy of the City of Pittsburgh, Department of City Planning.

\GistutorialHealth\PAGIS\StreetsCL.shp, courtesy of the City of Pittsburgh, Department of City Planning.

\GistutorialHealth\PAGIS\Walnut.jpg, used with permission from Kristen S. Kurland.

\GistutorialHealth\PAGIS\FifthForbes.jpg, used with permission from Kristen S. Kurland.

Tutorial 5 data sources include:

\GistutorialHealth\Pennsylvania\Copytr42_d00.shp, courtesy of U.S. Census Bureau TIGER.

Screen captures of www.census.gov, courtesy of the U.S. Census. All U.S. Census Bureau materials, regardless of the media, are entirely in the public domain. There are no user fees, site licenses, or any special agreements, etc., for the public or private use, and/or reuse of any census title. As a tax-funded product, it is all in the public record.

Screen captures of www.factfinder.census.gov, courtesy of the U.S. Census. All U.S. Census Bureau materials, regardless of the media, are entirely in the public domain. There are no user fees, site licenses, or any special agreements, etc., for the public or private use, and/or reuse of any census title. As a tax-funded product, it is all in the public record.

\GistutorialHealth\ACHD\Copy_dt_dec_2003_sf3_u_data1.xls, courtesy of U.S. Census Bureau; Census 2000, Summary File 3; generated by Kristen S. Kurland; using American FactFinder, http://factfinder.census.gov; (7 June 2005).

\GistutorialHealth\ACHD\Copy_YrBuilt.dbf, courtesy of U.S. Census Bureau; Census 2000, Summary File 3; generated by Kristen S. Kurland; using American FactFinder, http://factfinder.census.gov; (7 June 2005).

\GistutorialHealth\ACHD\copy_ccd0042003.zip, courtesy of U.S. Census Bureau TIGER.

\GistutorialHealth\ACHD\copy_lkB42003.zip,,courtesy of U.S. Census Bureau TIGER.

\GistutorialHealth\ACHD\copy_wat42003.zip, courtesy of U.S. Census Bureau TIGER.

\GistutorialHealth\ACHD\HousingComplaints.dbf, courtesy of Allegheny County Health Department.

\GistutorialHealth\ACHD\ElevatedBloodCases.dbf, courtesy of Allegheny County Health Department.

Tutorial 6 data sources include:

\GistutorialHealth\UnitedStates\ZipCodes.shp, from ESRI Data & Maps, 2005, courtesy of TANA/GDT, ESRI BIS (Pop2004 field).

\GistutorialHealth\UnitedStates\States.shp, from ESRI Data & Maps, 2007, courtesy of ArcUSA, U.S. Census, ESRI (Pop2005 field).

\GistutorialHealth\SiteSelection\Patients.dbf, fictitious database.

\GistutorialHealth\SiteSlection\TriStateZipCodes.shp, from ESRI Data & Maps, 2007, courtesy of Tele Atlas, ESRI (Pop2005 field).

\GistutorialHealth\UnitedStates\Counties.shp, from ESRI Data & Maps, 2007, courtesy of ArcUSA, U.S. Census, ESRI (Pop2005 field).

\GistutorialHealth\SiteSelection\TriStateCities.shp, from ESRI Data & Maps, 2004, courtesy of U.S. Census.

\GistutorialHealth\UnitedStates\Interstates.shp, from ESRI Data & Maps, 2004, courtesy of U.S. Bureau of Transportation Statistics.

\GistutorialHealth\SiteSelection\Streets.shp, courtesy of US Census Bureau TIGER.

\GistutorialHealth\SiteSelection\Hospitals.dbf, fictitious database.

\GistutorialHealth\SiteSelection\MammographyClinicsAlleghenyCountyPA.dbf, courtesy of U.S. Food and Drug Administration, Department of Health and Human Services.

\GistutorialHealth\Pennsylvania\PACounties.shp, from ESRI Data & Maps, 2007, courtesy of ArcUSA, U.S. Census, ESRI (Pop2005 field).

\GistutorialHealth\Pennsylvania\PATractsFemale40-60.shp, courtesy of U.S. Census Bureau TIGER.

Tutorial 7 data sources include:

\GistutorialHealth\PedestrianInjuries\InjuriesJones.shp, courtesy of the Children's Hospital of Pittsburgh.

\GistutorialHealth\PedestrianInjuries\InjuriesSmith.shp, courtesy of the Children's Hospital of Pittsburgh.

\GistutorialHealth\PedestrianInjuries\tgr42003lkA.shp, courtesy of U.S. Census Bureau TIGER.

\GistutorialHealth\PedestrianInjuries\tgr42003ccd00.shp, courtesy of U.S. Census Bureau TIGER.

\GistutorialHealth\PedestrianInjuries\tgr42003wat.shp, courtesy of U.S. Census Bureau TIGER.

\GistutorialHealth\PedestrianInjuries\tgr42003trt00.shp, courtesy of U.S. Census Bureau TIGER.

\GistutorialHealth\PAGIS\ParksPlaygrounds.shp, courtesy of the City of Pittsburgh, Department of City Planning.

\GistutorialHealth\PAGIS\Neighborhoods.shp, courtesy of the City of Pittsburgh, Department of City Planning.

\GistutorialHealth\PAGIS\BlockCentroids.shp, courtesy of U.S. Census Bureau TIGER.

\GistutorialHealth\PAGIS\Schools.shp, courtesy of the City of Pittsburgh, Department of City Planning.

\GistutorialHealth\PAGIS\ConvenienceStores.shp, courtesy of the Allegheny County Health Department.

\GistutorialHealth\SolutionComponents\Chapter7\InjuryResidences.shp, courtesy of the Children's Hospital of Pittsburgh.

Tutorial 8 data sources include:

\GistutorialHealth\Nebraska\Nebraska.shp, from ESRI Data & Maps, 2007, courtesy of ArcUSA, U.S. Census, ESRI (Pop2005 field).

\GistutorialHealth\Nebraska\NebraskaBlocks.shp, courtesy of U.S. Census Bureau TIGER.

\GistutorialHealth\UnitedStates\ZipCodes.shp, from ESRI Data & Maps, 2005, courtesy of TANA/GDT, ESRI BIS (Pop2004 field).

\GistutorialHealth\Nebraska\NebraskaCities.shp, from ESRI Data & Maps, 2004, courtesy of U.S. Census.

\GistutorialHealth\Nebraska\NebraskaHRR.shp, from The Dartmouth Atlas of Health Care, courtesy of The Trustees of Dartmouth College.

\GistutorialHealth\DouglasCounty\BlkGrpSF1.dbf, courtesy of U.S. Census.

\GistutorialHealth\DouglasCounty\BlkGrpSF3.dbf, courtesy of U.S. Census.

\GistutorialHealth\DouglasCounty\BlockCentroids.shp, courtesy of U.S. Census Bureau TIGER.

\GistutorialHealth\DouglasCounty\Blocks.shp, courtesy of U.S. Census Bureau TIGER.

\GistutorialHealth\DouglasCounty\ZipCodes.shp, from ESRI Data & Maps, 2004, courtesy of ESRI, derived from GDT, ESRI BIS (Pop2003 field).

\GistutorialHealth\SolutionComponents\Chapter8\BlockCentroids.shp, courtesy of U.S. Census Bureau TIGER

\GistutorialHealth\Nebraska\NebraskaHSA.shp, from The Dartmouth Atlas of Health Care, courtesy of The Trustees of Dartmouth College.

\GistutorialHealth\Massachusetts\Outline.shp, from ESRI Data & Maps, 2007, courtesy of ArcUSA, U.S. Census, ESRI (Pop2005 field).

\GistutorialHealth\Massachusetts\CensusBlocks.shp, courtesy of U.S. Census Bureau TIGER.

\GistutorialHealth\Massachusetts\UrbanAreas.shp, courtesy of U.S. Census.

\GistutorialHealth\Massachusetts\MajorCities.shp, from ESRI Data & Maps, 2004, courtesy of U.S. Census.

Tutorial 9 data sources include:

\Gistutorial\SpatialAnalyst\Zoning.shp, courtesy of the Allegheny County Division of Computer Services Geographic Information Systems Group.

 \Gistutorial\SpatialAnalyst\AllCoBlkGrps.shp, from ESRI Data & Maps, 2007, courtesy of Tele Atlas, U.S. Census, ESRI (Pop2005).

\Gistutorial\SpatialAnalyst\OHCA.shp, courtesy of Children's Hospital of Pittsburgh.

\Gistutorial\SpatialAnalyst\PennHills.shp, courtesy of U.S. Census Bureau TIGER.

\Gistutorial\SpatialAnalyst\Pittsburgh.shp, courtesy of U.S. Census Bureau TIGER.

\Gistutorial\SpatialAnalyst\Rivers.shp, courtesy of the U.S. Census Bureau.

\Gistutorial\SpatialAnalyst\Statistics.txt, courtesy of Wil Gorr, Carnegie Mellon University .

\Gistutorial\SpatialAnalyst\ZoningCommercialBuffer.shp, courtesy of Allegheny County Division of Computer Services Geographic Information Systems Group.

\Gistutorial\SpatialAnalyst\DEM, courtesy of U.S. Geological Survey, Department of the Interior/USGS.

\Gistutorial\SpatialAnalyst\LandUse, image courtesy of U.S. Geological Survey, Department of the Interior /USGS.

Tutorial 10 data sources include:

\GistutorialHealth\PAGIS\Neighborhood.shp, courtesy of the City of Pittsburgh, Department of City Planning.

\GistutorialHealth\PAGIS\StreetsCL.shp, courtesy of the City of Pittsburgh, Department of City Planning.

\GistutorialHealth\PAGIS\Sidewalks.shp, courtesy of the City of Pittsburgh, Department of City Planning.

\GistutorialHealth\PAGIS\Buildings.shp, courtesy of the City of Pittsburgh, Department of City Planning.

\GistutorialHealth\ACHD\PghFoodSources.dbf, courtesy of Allegheny County Health Department.

\GistutorialHealth\ACHD\OutbreakResidences.dbf, fictitious database.

\GistutorialHealth\ACHD\OutbreakWorkLocations.dbf, fictitious database.

\GistutorialHealth\PAGIS\BlockCentroids.shp, courtesy of U.S. Census TIGER.

\GistutorialHealth\PAGIS\FemaFlood.shp, courtesy of the City of Pittsburgh, Department of City Planning.

Tutorial 11 data sources include:

\GistutorialHealth\UnitedStates\States.shp, from ESRI Data & Maps, 2007, courtesy of ArcUSA, U.S. Census, ESRI (Pop2005 field).

\GistutorialHealth\ACHE\ACHEMembers.dbf, courtesy of the American College of Healthcare Executives.

\GistutorialHealth\ACHE\HEG_WHEN.shp, courtesy of the American College of Healthcare Executives.

\GistutorialHealth\UnitedStates\ZipCodes.shp, from ESRI Data & Maps, 2005, courtesy of TANA/GDT, ESRI BIS (Pop2004 field).

\GistutorialHealth\ACHE\GroupsDistricts1_2_3.dbf, courtesy of the American College of Healthcare Executives.

\GistutorialHealth\ACHE\GroupsDistricts4_5_6.dbf, courtesy of the American College of Healthcare Executives.

\GistutorialHealth\ACHE\ResolvedPartners.dbf, courtesy of the American College of Healthcare Executives.

Appendix B

Data license agreement

Important:

Read carefully before opening the sealed media package

ENVIRONMENTAL SYSTEMS RESEARCH INSTITUTE, INC. (ESRI), IS WILLING TO LICENSE THE ENCLOSED DATA AND RELATED MATERIALS TO YOU ONLY UPON THE CONDITION THAT YOU ACCEPT ALL OF THE TERMS AND CONDITIONS CONTAINED IN THIS LICENSE AGREEMENT. PLEASE READ THE TERMS AND CONDITIONS CAREFULLY BEFORE OPENING THE SEALED MEDIA PACKAGE. BY OPENING THE SEALED MEDIA PACKAGE, YOU ARE INDICATING YOUR ACCEPTANCE OF THE ESRI LICENSE AGREEMENT. IF YOU DO NOT AGREE TO THE TERMS AND CONDITIONS AS STATED, THEN ESRI IS UNWILLING TO LICENSE THE DATA AND RELATED MATERIALS TO YOU. IN SUCH EVENT, YOU SHOULD RETURN THE MEDIA PACKAGE WITH THE SEAL UNBROKEN AND ALL OTHER COMPONENTS TO ESRI.

ESRI License Agreement

This is a license agreement, and not an agreement for sale, between you (Licensee) and Environmental Systems Research Institute, Inc. (ESRI). This ESRI License Agreement (Agreement) gives Licensee certain limited rights to use the data and related materials (Data and Related Materials). All rights not specifically granted in this Agreement are reserved to ESRI and its Licensors.

Reservation of Ownership and Grant of License: ESRI and its Licensors retain exclusive rights, title, and ownership to the copy of the Data and Related Materials licensed under this Agreement and, hereby, grant to Licensee a personal, nonexclusive, nontransferable, royalty-free, worldwide license to use the Data and Related Materials based on the terms and conditions of this Agreement. Licensee agrees to use reasonable effort to protect the Data and Related Materials from unauthorized use, reproduction, distribution, or publication.

Proprietary Rights and Copyright: Licensee acknowledges that the Data and Related Materials are proprietary and confidential property of ESRI and its Licensors and are protected by United States copyright laws and applicable international copyright treaties and/or conventions.

Permitted Uses: Licensee may install the Data and Related Materials onto permanent storage device(s) for Licensee's own internal use.

Licensee may make only one (1) copy of the original Data and Related Materials for archival purposes during the term of this Agreement unless the right to make additional copies is granted to Licensee in writing by ESRI.

Licensee may internally use the Data and Related Materials provided by ESRI for the stated purpose of GIS training and education.

Uses Not Permitted: Licensee shall not sell, rent, lease, sublicense, lend, assign, time-share, or transfer, in whole or in part, or provide unlicensed Third Parties access to the Data and Related Materials or portions of the Data and Related Materials, any updates, or Licensee's rights under this Agreement.

Licensee shall not remove or obscure any copyright or trademark notices of ESRI or its Licensors.

Term and Termination: The license granted to Licensee by this Agreement shall commence upon the acceptance of this Agreement and shall continue until such time that Licensee elects in writing to discontinue use of the Data or Related Materials and terminates this Agreement. The Agreement shall automatically terminate without notice if Licensee fails to comply with any provision of this Agreement. Licensee shall then return to ESRI the Data and Related Materials. The parties hereby agree that all provisions that operate to protect the rights of ESRI and its Licensors shall remain in force should breach occur.

Disclaimer of Warranty: The Data and Related Materials contained herein are provided "as-is," without warranty of any kind, either express or implied, including, but not limited to, the implied warranties of merchantability, fitness for a particular purpose, or noninfringement. ESRI does not warrant that the Data and Related Materials will meet Licensee's needs or expectations, that the use of the Data and Related Materials will be uninterrupted, or that all nonconformities, defects, or errors can or will be corrected. ESRI is not inviting reliance on the Data or Related Materials for commercial planning or analysis purposes, and Licensee should always check actual data.

Data Disclaimer: The Data used herein has been derived from actual spatial or tabular information. In some cases, ESRI has manipulated and applied certain assumptions, analyses, and opinions to the Data solely for educational training purposes. Assumptions, analyses, opinions applied, and actual outcomes may vary. Again, ESRI is not inviting reliance on this Data, and the Licensee should always verify actual Data and exercise their own professional judgment when interpreting any outcomes.

Limitation of Liability: ESRI shall not be liable for direct, indirect, special, incidental, or consequential damages related to Licensee's use of the Data and Related Materials, even if ESRI is advised of the possibility of such damage.

No Implied Waivers: No failure or delay by ESRI or its Licensors in enforcing any right or remedy under this Agreement shall be construed as a waiver of any future or other exercise of such right or remedy by ESRI or its Licensors.

Order for Precedence: Any conflict between the terms of this Agreement and any FAR, DFAR, purchase order, or other terms shall be resolved in favor of the terms expressed in this Agreement, subject to the government's minimum rights unless agreed otherwise.

Export Regulation: Licensee acknowledges that this Agreement and the performance thereof are subject to compliance with any and all applicable United States laws, regulations, or orders relating to the export of data thereto. Licensee agrees to comply with all laws, regulations, and orders of the United States in regard to any export of such technical data.

Severability: If any provision(s) of this Agreement shall be held to be invalid, illegal, or unenforceable by a court or other tribunal of competent jurisdiction, the validity, legality, and enforceability of the remaining provisions shall not in any way be affected or impaired thereby.

Governing Law: This Agreement, entered into in the County of San Bernardino, shall be construed and enforced in accordance with and be governed by the laws of the United States of America and the State of California without reference to conflict of laws principles. The parties hereby consent to the personal jurisdiction of the courts of this county and waive their rights to change venue.

Entire Agreement: The parties agree that this Agreement constitutes the sole and entire agreement of the parties as to the matter set forth herein and supersedes any previous agreements, understandings, and arrangements between the parties relating hereto.

Appendix C

Installing the data and software

GIS Tutorial for Health includes one DVD with exercise data and one DVD with ArcGIS Desktop (ArcView license, single-use, 180-day trial) software. You will find both in the back of this book. Installation of the exercise data DVD takes approximately five minutes and requires around 556 MB of hard-disk space. Installation of the ArcGIS Desktop software DVD with extensions takes approximately 25 minutes and requires at least 2.4 GB of hard-disk space. Installation times will vary with your computer's speed and available memory.

If you previously installed data for an earlier edition of *GIS Tutorial for Health*, you cannot simply copy the current data over it. You must uninstall the previous data before you install the exercise data that comes with this book.

If you already have a licensed copy of ArcGIS Desktop installed on your computer (or accessible through a network), do not install the software DVD. Use your licensed software to do the exercises in this book. If you have an older version of ArcGIS installed on your computer, you must uninstall it before you can install the software DVD that comes with this book.

The exercises in this book work only with ArcGIS 9.3 or higher.

Installing the exercise data

Follow the steps below to install the exercise data.

1   Put the data CD in your computer's CD drive. A splash screen will appear.

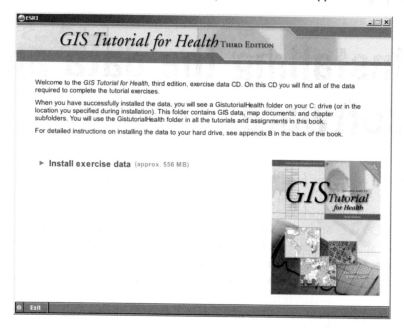

2   Read the welcome, then click the Install exercise data link. This launches the Setup wizard.

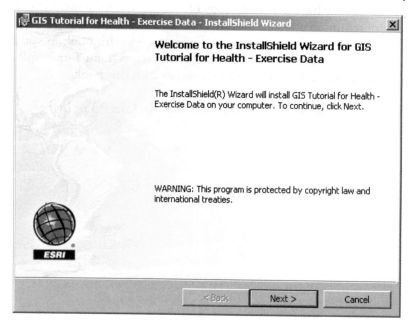

3   Click Next. Read and accept the license agreement terms, then click Next.

4 Accept the default installation folder. We recommend that you do not choose an alternative location.

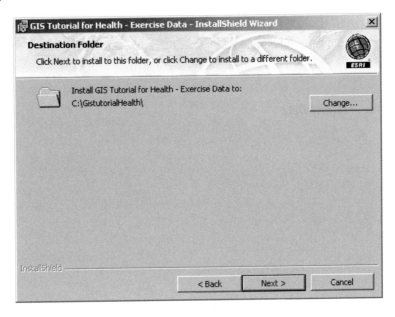

5 Click Next. The installation will take a few moments. When the installation is complete, you will see the following message:

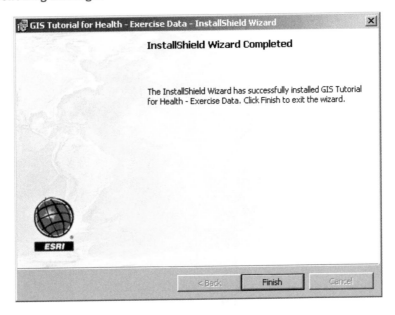

6 Click Finish. The exercise data is installed on your computer in a folder called GistutorialHealth.

Uninstalling the exercise data

To uninstall the exercise data from your computer, open your operating system's control panel and double-click the Add/Remove Programs icon. In the Add/Remove Programs dialog box, select the following entry and follow the prompts to remove it:

GIS Tutorial for Health - Exercise Data

Installing the software

The ArcGIS software included on this DVD is intended for educational purposes only. Once installed and registered, the software will run for 180 days. The software cannot be reinstalled nor can the time limit be extended. It is recommended that you uninstall this software when it expires.

Follow the steps below to install the software.

1 **Put the software DVD in your computer's DVD drive. A splash screen will appear.**

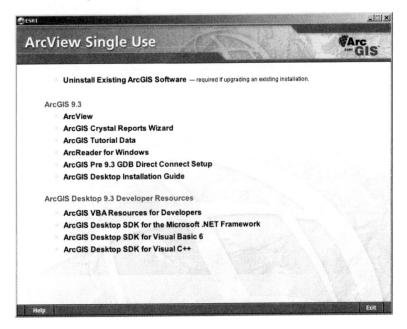

2 **Click the ArcGIS ArcView installation option. On the startup window, click Install ArcGIS Desktop. This will launch the Setup wizard.**

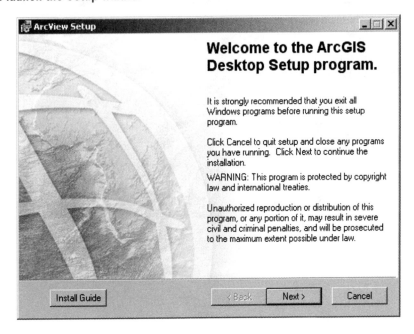

3 Read the Welcome, then click Next.

4 Read the license agreement. Click "I accept the license agreement" and click Next.

5 The default installation type is Typical, which is the one that is needed for this install. Click Next.

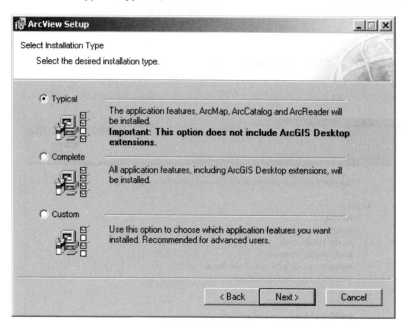

6 Click Next. Accept the default installation folder or click Browse and navigate to the drive or folder location where you want to install the software.

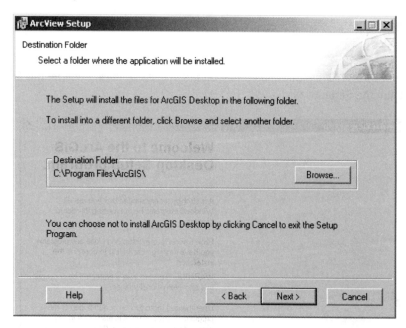

7   Click Next. Accept the default installation folder or navigate to the drive or folder where you want to install Python, a scripting language used by some ArcGIS geoprocessing functions. (You won't see this panel if you already have Python installed.) We recommend that you accept the default folder. Click Next.

8   The installation paths for ArcGIS and Python are confirmed. Click Next. The software will take several minutes to install on your computer. When the installation is finished, you see the following message:

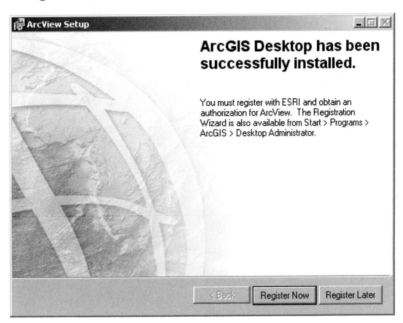

9   Click Register Now and follow the registration process. The registration code is located at the bottom of the software DVD jacket in the back of the book.

If you have questions or encounter problems during the installation process or while using this book, please use the resources listed below. (The ESRI Technical Support Department does not answer questions regarding the ArcGIS software DVD, the *GIS Tutorial for Health* exercise data CD, or the contents of the book itself.)

•   To resolve problems with the trial software or exercise data, or to report mistakes in the book, send an e-mail to ESRI workbook support at learngis@esri.com.

•   To stay informed about exercise updates, FAQs, and errata, visit the book's Web page at www.esri.com/esripress/gistutorialhealth3.

Uninstalling the software

To uninstall the software from your computer, open your operating system's control panel and double-click the Add/Remove Programs icon. In the Add/Remove Programs dialog box, select the following entry and follow the prompts to remove it:

ArcGIS Desktop

Related titles from ESRI Press

GIS Tutorial, Third Edition
ISBN 978-1-58948-205-0

GIS Tutorial for Marketing
ISBN 978-1-58948-079-7

Getting to Know ArcView GIS
ISBN 978-1-879102-46-0

GIS Tutorial for Homeland Security
ISBN 978-1-58948-188-6

Getting to Know ArcGIS Desktop, Second Edition, Updated for ArcGIS 9.3
ISBN 978-1-58948-210-4

GIS for Everyone, Third Edition
ISBN 978-1-58948-056-8

ESRI Press publishes books about the science, application, and technology of GIS. Ask for these titles at your local bookstore or order by calling 1-800-447-9778. You can also read book descriptions, read reviews, and shop online at www.esri.com/esripress. Outside the United States, contact your local ESRI distributor.